BLACKWELL

UNDERGROUND CLINICAL VIGNETTES

BEHAVIORAL SCIENCE, 4E

BLACKWELL

UNDERGROUND CLINICAL VIGNETTES

BEHAVIORAL SCIENCE, 4E

VIKAS BHUSHAN, MD
Series Editor
University of California, San Francisco, Class of 1991
Diagnostic Radiologist

VISHAL PALL, MD MPH
Series Editor
Internist and Preventive Medicine Specialist
Government Medical College, Chandigarh – Panjab University – India, Class of 1997
Graduate School of Biomedical Sciences at UTMB Galveston, MPH, Class of 2004

TAO LE, MD
University of California, San Francisco, Class of 1996

HOANG NGUYEN, MD, MBA
Northwestern University, Class of 2001

JOSEPH HASTINGS
David Geffen School of Medicine at UCLA/ Class of 2006
UCLA School of Public Health, MPH/ Class of 2006

POURYA M.GHAZI, MD
Senior Fellow, Department of Laboratory Medicine/ University of Washington, Seattle

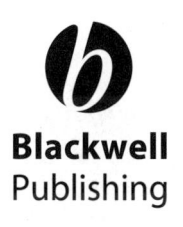

Blackwell
Publishing

WM
18.2
B4185
2005

© 2005 by Blackwell Publishing

Blackwell Publishing, Inc., 350 Main Street, Malden, Massachusetts 02148-5018, USA
Blackwell Publishing Ltd, 9600 Garsington Road, Oxford OX4 2DQ, UK
Blackwell Publishing Asia Pty Ltd, 550 Swanston Street, Carlton, Victoria 3053, Australia

All rights reserved. No part of this publication may be reproduced in any form or by any electronic or mechanical means, including information storage and retrieval systems, without permission in writing from the publisher, except by a reviewer who may quote brief passages in a review.

05 06 07 08 5 4 3 2 1

ISBN-13: 978-1-4051-0410-4
ISBN-10: 1-4051-0410-4

Library of Congress Cataloging-in-Publication Data

Behavioral science / Vikhas Bhushan . . . [et al.].— 4th ed.
   p. ; cm. — (Blackwell underground clinical vignettes)
   ISBN-13: 978-1-4051-0410-4 (pbk. : alk. paper)
   ISBN-10: 1-4051-0410-4 (pbk. : alk. paper) 1. Psychiatry—Case studies. 2. Neuropsychiatry—Case studies. 3. Behavioral sciences—Case studies. 4. Psychiatry—Examinations, questions, etc. 5. Neuropsychiatry—Examinations, questions, etc. 6. Behavioral sciences—Examinations, questions, etc. 7. Physicians—Licenses—United States—Examinations—Study guides.
   [DNLM: 1. Behavioral Symptoms—diagnosis—Case Reports. 2. Behavioral Symptoms—diagnosis—Problems and Exercises. 3. Behavioral Symptoms—therapy—Case Reports. 4. Behavioral Symptoms—therapy—Problems and Exercises. WM 18.2 B4185 2005] I. Bhushan, Vikas. II. Series: Blackwell's underground clinical vignettes.

RC465.B5259 2005
616.89′0076—dc22

2005003546

A catalogue record for this title is available from the British Library

Acquisitions: Nancy Anastasi Duffy
Development/Production: Jennifer Kowalewski
Cover and Interior design: Leslie Haimes
Typesetter: Graphicraft in Quarry Bay, Hong Kong
Printed and bound by Capital City Press in Berlin, VT

For further information on Blackwell Publishing, visit our website:
www.blackwellmedstudent.com

NOTICE

The indications and dosages of all drugs in this book have been recommended in the medical literature and conform to the practices of the general community. The medications described do not necessarily have specific approval by the Food and Drug Administration for use in the diseases and dosages for which they are recommended. The package insert for each drug should be consulted for use and dosage as approved by the FDA. Because standards for usage change, it is advisable to keep abreast of revised recommendations, particularly those concerning new drugs.

The authors of this volume have taken care that the information contained herein is accurate and compatible with the standards generally accepted at the time of publication. Nevertheless, it is difficult to ensure that all the information given is entirely accurate for all circumstances. The publisher and authors do not guarantee the contents of this book and disclaim any liability, loss, or damage incurred as a consequence, directly or indirectly, of the use and application of any of the contents of this volume.

The publisher's policy is to use permanent paper from mills that operate a sustainable forestry policy, and which has been manufactured from pulp processed using acid-free and elementary chlorine-free practices. Furthermore, the publisher ensures that the text paper and cover board used have met acceptable environmental accreditation standards.

CONTENTS

CONTRIBUTORS ix
ACKNOWLEDGMENTS x
HOW TO USE THIS BOOK xii
ABBREVIATIONS xiii

NEUROLOGY

Case 1	1
Case 2	2
Case 3	3
Case 4	4
Case 5	5
Case 6	6
Case 7	7
Case 8	8
Case 9	9
Case 10	10
Case 11	11
Case 12	12

DEFENSE MECHANISM

Case 13	13
Case 14	14
Case 15	15
Case 16	16
Case 17	17
Case 18	18
Case 19	19
Case 20	20
Case 21	21
Case 22	22
Case 23	23
Case 24	24
Case 25	25

ADJUSTMENT DISORDERS

Case 26	26

ANXIETY DISORDERS

Case 27	27
Case 28	28
Case 29	29
Case 30	30
Case 31	31

CHILD PSYCHIATRY

Case 32	32
Case 33	33
Case 34	34
Case 35	35
Case 36	36
Case 37	37
Case 38	38
Case 39	39
Case 40	40

DISSOCIATIVE IDENTITY DISORDER

Case 41	41
Case 42	42
Case 43	43
Case 44	44

EATING DISORDERS

Case 45	45
Case 46	46

FACTITIOUS DISORDERS

Case 47	47
Case 48	48

GENDER IDENTITY DISORDER

Case 49	49

MOOD DISORDERS

Case 50	50
Case 51	51

Case 52	52
Case 53	53
Case 54	54
Case 55	55
Case 56	56
Case 57	57
Case 58	58
Case 59	59

PARAPHILIA

Case 60	60
Case 61	61
Case 62	62
Case 63	63
Case 64	64
Case 65	65

PERSONALITY DISORDERS

Case 66	66
Case 67	67
Case 68	68
Case 69	69
Case 70	70
Case 71	71
Case 72	72
Case 73	73
Case 74	74
Case 75	75
Case 76	76

PSYCHOTIC DISORDERS

Case 77	77
Case 78	78
Case 79	79
Case 80	80
Case 81	81
Case 82	82

Case 83	83
Case 84	84
Case 85	85

SLEEP DISORDERS

Case 86	86
Case 87	87

SOMATOFORM DISORDERS

Case 88	88
Case 89	89
Case 90	90
Case 91	91
Case 92	92
Case 93	93
Case 94	94
Case 95	95

PSYCHOPHARMACOLOGY

Case 96	96
Case 97	97

ANSWER KEY	99
Q&AS	101

CONTRIBUTORS

Bahar Sedarati, MD
Shiraz University School of Medicine, Class of 1995
Associate Professor, Department of Pathology, St. Luke's University School of Medicine

Chad Silverberg
Philadelphia College of Osteopathic Medicine, Class of 2004
Resident in Internal Medicine, Cleveland Clinic Foundation
Radiology Resident, Christiana Hospital (From 2005)

Ishnella Azad, MD
University of California Los Angeles
Resident in Psychiatry

Kaushik Mukherjee
David Geffen School of Medicine at UCLA, Class of 2005

Kyong Un Chong
Joan C. Edwards School of Medicine, West Virginia, Class of 2005

Matthew Y.C. Lin
David Geffen School of Medicine at UCLA, Class of 2005

Monika Gupta MD
Kasturba Medical College – Manipal Academy of Higher Education, Class of 2002

Mustaqeem A Siddiqui, MD
Aga Khan University Medical College, Class of 2002
Resident in Internal Medicine, Mayo Clinic, Rochester MN

Siddarth Shah, MD
Mt. Sinai School of Medicine, New York
Resident in Preventive and Community Education

Sunit Das, MD
Northwestern University, Class of 2000
Faculty Reviewer

Rita Joshi, MD
University of California Los Angeles
Attending Physician in Psychiatry

ACKNOWLEDGMENTS

Throughout the production of this book, we have had the support of many friends and colleagues. Special thanks to our support team including Andrea Fellows, Anastasia Anderson, Srishti Gupta, Anu Gupta, Mona Pall, Jonathan Kirsch and Chirag Amin. For prior contributions we thank Gianni Le Nguyen, Tarun Mathur, Alex Grimm, Sonia Santos and Elizabeth Sanders.

For submitting comments, corrections, editing, proofreading, and assistance across all of the vignette titles in all editions, we collectively thank:

Tara Adamovich, Carolyn Alexander, Kris Alden, Henry E. Aryan, Lynman Bacolor, Natalie Barteneva, Dean Bartholomew, Debashish Behera, Sumit Bhatia, Sanjay Bindra, Dave Brinton, Julianne Brown, Alexander Brownie, Tamara Callahan, David Canes, Bryan Casey, Aaron Caughey, Hebert Chen, Jonathan Cheng, Arnold Cheung, Arnold Chin, Simion Chiosea, Yoon Cho, Samuel Chung, Gretchen Conant, Vladimir Coric, Christopher Cosgrove, Ronald Cowan, Karekin R. Cunningham, A. Sean Dalley, Rama Dandamudi, Sunit Das, Ryan Armando Dave, John David, Emmanuel de la Cruz, Robert DeMello, Navneet Dhillon, Sharmila Dissanaike, David Donson, Adolf Etchegaray, Alea Eusebio, Priscilla A. Frase, David Frenz, Kristin Gaumer, Yohannes Gebreegziabher, Anil Gehi, Tony George, L.M. Gotanco, Parul Goyal, Alexander Grimm, Rajeev Gupta, Ahmad Halim, Sue Hall, David Hasselbacher, Tamra Heimert, Michelle Higley, Dan Hoit, Eric Jackson, Tim Jackson, Sundar Jayaraman, Pei-Ni Jone, Aarchan Joshi, Rajni K. Jutla, Faiyaz Kapadi, Seth Karp, Aaron S. Kesselheim, Sana Khan, Andrew Pin-wei Ko, Francis Kong, Paul Konitzky, Warren S. Krackov, Benjamin H.S. Lau, Ann LaCasce, Connie Lee, Scott Lee, Guillermo Lehmann, Kevin Leung, Paul Levett, Warren Levinson, Eric Ley, Ken Lin, Pavel Lobanov, J. Mark Maddox, Aram Mardian, Samir Mehta, Gil Melmed, Joe Messina, Robert Mosca, Michael Murphy, Vivek Nandkarni, Siva Naraynan, Carvell Nguyen, Linh Nguyen, Deanna Nobleza, Craig Nodurft, George Noumi, Darin T. Okuda, Adam L. Palance, Paul Pamphrus, Jinha Park, Sonny Patel, Ricardo Pietrobon, Riva L. Rahl, Aashita Randeria, Rachan Reddy, Beatriu Reig, Marilou Reyes, Jeremy Richmon, Tai Roe, Rick Roller, Rajiv Roy, Diego Ruiz, Anthony Russell, Sanjay Sahgal, Urmimala Sarkar, John Schilling, Isabell Schmitt, Daren Schuhmacher, Sonal Shah, Fadi Abu Shahin, Edie Shen, Justin Smith, John Stulak, Lillian Su, Julie Sundaram, Rita Suri, Seth Sweetser, Antonio Talayero, Merita Tan, Mark Tanaka, Eric Taylor, Jess Thompson, Indi Trehan, Raymond Turner, Okafo Uchenna, Eric Uyguanco, Richa Varma, John Wages, Alan Wang, Eunice Wang, Andy Weiss, Amy Williams, Brian Yang, Hany Zaky, Ashraf Zaman and David Zipf.

Please let us know if your name has been missed or misspelled and we will be happy to make the update in the next edition.

For generously contributing images to the entire Underground Clinical Vignette Step 1 series, we collectively thank the staff at Blackwell Publishing in Oxford, Boston, and Berlin as well as:

- Axford, J. Medicine. Osney Mead: Blackwell Science Ltd, 1996. Figures 2.14, 2.15, 2.16, 2.27, 2.28, 2.31, 2.35, 2.36, 2.38, 2.43, 2.65a, 2.65b, 2.65c, 2.103b, 2.105b, 3.20b, 3.21, 8.27, 8.27b, 8.77b, 8.77c, 10.81b, 10.96a, 12.28a, 14.6, 14.16, 14.50.

- Bannister B, Begg N, Gillespie S. Infectious Disease, 2nd Edition. Osney Mead: Blackwell Science Ltd, 2000. Figures 2.8, 3.4, 5.28, 18.10, W5.32, W5.6.

- Berg D. Advanced Clinical Skills and Physical Diagnosis. Blackwell Science Ltd., 1999. Figures 7.10, 7.12, 7.13, 7.2, 7.3, 7.7, 7.8, 7.9, 8.1, 8.2, 8.4, 8.5, 9.2, 10.2, 11.3, 11.5, 12.6.

- Cuschieri A, Hennessy TPJ, Greenhalgh RM, Rowley DA, Grace PA. Clinical Surgery. Osney Mead: Blackwell Science Ltd, 1996. Figures 13.19, 18.22, 18.33.

- Gillespie SH, Bamford K. *Medical Microbiology and Infection at a Glance.* Osney Mead.: Blackwell Science Ltd, 2000, Figures 20, 23.

- Ginsberg L. Lecture Notes on Neurology, 7th Edition. Osney Mead: Blackwell Science Ltd, 1999. Figures 12.3, 18.3, 18.3b.

- Elliott T, Hastings M, Desselberger U. Lecture Notes on Medical Microbiology, 3rd Edition. Osney Mead: Blackwell Science Ltd, 1997. Figures 2, 5, 7, 8, 9, 11, 12, 14, 15, 16, 17, 19, 20, 25, 26, 27, 29, 30, 34, 35, 52.

- Mehta AB, Hoffbrand AV. Haematology at a Glance. Osney Mead: Blackwell Science Ltd, 2000. Figures 22.1, 22.2, 22.3.

HOW TO USE THIS BOOK

This series was originally developed to address the increasing number of clinical vignette questions on medical examinations, including the USMLE Step 1 and Step 2.

Each UCV 1 book uses a series of approximately 100 "**supra-prototypical**" **cases as a way to condense testable facts and associations**. The clinical vignettes in this series are designed to give added emphasis to pathogenesis, epidemiology, management and complications. Although each case tends to present all the signs, symptoms, and diagnostic findings for a particular illness, **patients generally will not present with such a "complete" picture either clinically or on a medical examination**. Cases are not meant to simulate a potential real patient or an exam vignette. **All the boldfaced "buzzwords" are for learning purposes** and are not necessarily expected to be found in any one patient with the disease.

Definitions of selected important terms are placed within the vignettes in (small caps) in parentheses. Other parenthetical remarks often refer to the pathophysiology or mechanism of disease. The format should also help students learn to present cases succinctly during oral "bullet" presentations on clinical rotations. The cases are meant to serve as a condensed review, not as a primary reference. The information provided in this book has been prepared with a great deal of thought and careful research. This book should not, however, be considered as your sole source of information. Corrections, suggestions and submissions of new cases are encouraged and will be acknowledged and incorporated when appropriate in future editions.

We hope that you find the *Blackwell Underground Clinical Vignettes* series informative and useful. We welcome feedback and suggestions you have about this book, or any published by Blackwell Publishing.

Please e-mail us at medfeedback@bos.blackwellpublishing.com.

ABBREVIATIONS

ABGs	arterial blood gases
ABPA	allergic bronchopulmonary aspergillosis
ACA	anticardiolipin antibody
ACE	angiotensin-converting enzyme
ACL	anterior cruciate ligament
ACTH	adrenocorticotropic hormone
AD	adjustment disorder
ADA	adenosine deaminase
ADD	attention deficit disorder
ADH	antidiuretic hormone
ADHD	attention deficit hyperactivity disorder
ADP	adenosine diphosphate
AFO	ankle-foot orthosis
AFP	α-fetoprotein
AIDS	acquired immunodeficiency syndrome
ALL	acute lymphocytic leukemia
ALS	amyotrophic lateral sclerosis
ALT	alanine aminotransferase
AML	acute myelogenous leukemia
ANA	antinuclear antibody
Angio	angiography
AP	anteroposterior
APKD	adult polycystic kidney disease
aPTT	activated partial thromboplastin time
ARDS	adult respiratory distress syndrome
5-ASA	5-aminosalicylic acid
ASCA	antibodies to *Saccharomyces cerevisiae*
ASO	antistreptolysin O
AST	aspartate aminotransferase
ATLL	adult T-cell leukemia/lymphoma
ATPase	adenosine triphosphatase
AV	arteriovenous, atrioventricular
AZT	azidothymidine (zidovudine)
BAL	British antilewisite (dimercaprol)
BCG	bacille Calmette-Guérin
BE	barium enema
BP	blood pressure
BPH	benign prostatic hypertrophy
BUN	blood urea nitrogen
CABG	coronary artery bypass grafting
CAD	coronary artery disease
CaEDTA	calcium edetate
CALLA	common acute lymphoblastic leukemia antigen
cAMP	cyclic adenosine monophosphate
C-ANCA	cytoplasmic antineutrophil cytoplasmic antibody
CBC	complete blood count

CBD	common bile duct
CCU	cardiac care unit
CD	cluster of differentiation
2-CdA	2-chlorodeoxyadenosine
CEA	carcinoembryonic antigen
CFTR	cystic fibrosis transmembrane conductance regulator
cGMP	cyclic guanosine monophosphate
CHF	congestive heart failure
CK	creatine kinase
CK-MB	creatine kinase, MB fraction
CLL	chronic lymphocytic leukemia
CML	chronic myelogenous leukemia
CMV	cytomegalovirus
CN	cranial nerve
CNS	central nervous system
COPD	chronic obstructive pulmonary disease
COX	cyclooxygenase
CP	cerebellopontine
CPAP	continuous positive airway pressure
CPK	creatine phosphokinase
CPPD	calcium pyrophosphate dihydrate
CPR	cardiopulmonary resuscitation
CREST	calcinosis, Raynaud's phenomenon, esophageal involvement, sclerodactyly, telangiectasia (syndrome)
CRP	C-reactive protein
CSF	cerebrospinal fluid
CSOM	chronic suppurative otitis media
CT	cardiac transplant, computed tomography
CVA	cerebrovascular accident
CXR	chest x-ray
d4T	didehydrodeoxythymidine (stavudine)
DCS	decompression sickness
DDH	developmental dysplasia of the hip
ddI	dideoxyinosine (didanosine)
DES	diethylstilbestrol
DEXA	dual-energy x-ray absorptiometry
DHEAS	dehydroepiandrosterone sulfate
DIC	disseminated intravascular coagulation
DIF	direct immunofluorescence
DIP	distal interphalangeal (joint)
DKA	diabetic ketoacidosis
DL_{CO}	diffusing capacity of carbon monoxide
DMSA	2,3-dimercaptosuccinic acid
DNA	deoxyribonucleic acid
DNase	deoxyribonuclease
2,3-DPG	2,3-diphosphoglycerate

dsDNA	double-stranded DNA
DSM	Diagnostic and Statistical Manual
dsRNA	double-stranded RNA
DTP	diphtheria, tetanus, pertussis (vaccine)
DTPA	diethylenetriamine-penta-acetic acid
DTs	delirium tremens
DVT	deep venous thrombosis
EBV	Epstein-Barr virus
ECG	electrocardiography
Echo	echocardiography
ECM	erythema chronicum migrans
ECT	electroconvulsive therapy
EEG	electroencephalography
EF	ejection fraction, elongation factor
EGD	esophagogastroduodenoscopy
EHEC	enterohemorrhagic *E. coli*
EIA	enzyme immunoassay
ELISA	enzyme-linked immunosorbent assay
EM	electron microscopy
EMG	electromyography
ENT	ears, nose, and throat
EPVE	early prosthetic valve endocarditis
ER	emergency room
ERCP	endoscopic retrograde cholangiopancreatography
ERT	estrogen replacement therapy
ESR	erythrocyte sedimentation rate
ETEC	enterotoxigenic *E. coli*
EtOH	ethanol
FAP	familial adenomatous polyposis
FEV_1	forced expiratory volume in 1 second
FH	familial hypercholesterolemia
FNA	fine-needle aspiration
FSH	follicle-stimulating hormone
FTA-ABS	fluorescent treponemal antibody absorption test
FVC	forced vital capacity
G6PD	glucose-6-phosphate dehydrogenase
GABA	gamma-aminobutyric acid
GERD	gastroesophageal reflux disease
GFR	glomerular filtration rate
GGT	gamma-glutamyltransferase
GH	growth hormone
GI	gastrointestinal
GnRH	gonadotropin-releasing hormone
GU	genitourinary
GVHD	graft-versus-host disease
HAART	highly active antiretroviral therapy

HAV	hepatitis A virus
Hb	hemoglobin
HbA-1C	hemoglobin A-1C
HBsAg	hepatitis B surface antigen
HBV	hepatitis B virus
hCG	human chorionic gonadotropin
HCO_3	bicarbonate
Hct	hematocrit
HCV	hepatitis C virus
HDL	high-density lipoprotein
HDL-C	high-density lipoprotein-cholesterol
HEENT	head, eyes, ears, nose, and throat (exam)
HELLP	hemolysis, elevated LFTs, low platelets (syndrome)
HFMD	hand, foot, and mouth disease
HGPRT	hypoxanthine-guanine phosphoribosyltransferase
5-HIAA	5-hydroxyindoleacetic acid
HIDA	hepato-iminodiacetic acid (scan)
HIV	human immunodeficiency virus
HLA	human leukocyte antigen
HMG-CoA	hydroxymethylglutaryl-coenzyme A
HMP	hexose monophosphate
HPI	history of present illness
HPV	human papillomavirus
HR	heart rate
HRIG	human rabies immune globulin
HRS	hepatorenal syndrome
HRT	hormone replacement therapy
HSG	hysterosalpingography
HSV	herpes simplex virus
HTLV	human T-cell leukemia virus
HUS	hemolytic-uremic syndrome
HVA	homovanillic acid
ICP	intracranial pressure
ICU	intensive care unit
ID/CC	identification and chief complaint
IDDM	insulin-dependent diabetes mellitus
IFA	immunofluorescent antibody
Ig	immunoglobulin
IGF	insulin-like growth factor
IHSS	idiopathic hypertrophic subaortic stenosis
IM	intramuscular
IMA	inferior mesenteric artery
INH	isoniazid
INR	International Normalized Ratio
IP_3	inositol 1,4,5-triphosphate
IPF	idiopathic pulmonary fibrosis

ITP	idiopathic thrombocytopenic purpura
IUD	intrauterine device
IV	intravenous
IVC	inferior vena cava
IVIG	intravenous immunoglobulin
IVP	intravenous pyelography
JRA	juvenile rheumatoid arthritis
JVP	jugular venous pressure
KOH	potassium hydroxide
KUB	kidney, ureter, bladder
LCM	lymphocytic choriomeningitis
LDH	lactate dehydrogenase
LDL	low-density lipoprotein
LE	lupus erythematosus (cell)
LES	lower esophageal sphincter
LFTs	liver function tests
LH	luteinizing hormone
LMN	lower motor neuron
LP	lumbar puncture
LPVE	late prosthetic valve endocarditis
L/S	lecithin-sphingomyelin (ratio)
LSD	lysergic acid diethylamide
LT	labile toxin
LV	left ventricular
LVH	left ventricular hypertrophy
Lytes	electrolytes
Mammo	mammography
MAO	monoamine oxidase (inhibitor)
MCP	metacarpophalangeal (joint)
MCTD	mixed connective tissue disorder
MCV	mean corpuscular volume
MEN	multiple endocrine neoplasia
MI	myocardial infarction
MIBG	meta-iodobenzylguanidine (radioisotope)
MMR	measles, mumps, rubella (vaccine)
MPGN	membranoproliferative glomerulonephritis
MPS	mucopolysaccharide
MPTP	1-methyl-4-phenyl-tetrahydropyridine
MR	magnetic resonance (imaging)
mRNA	messenger ribonucleic acid
MRSA	methicillin-resistant *S. aureus*
MTP	metatarsophalangeal (joint)
NAD	nicotinamide adenine dinucleotide
NADP	nicotinamide adenine dinucleotide phosphate
NADPH	reduced nicotinamide adenine dinucleotide phosphate
NF	neurofibromatosis

NIDDM	non-insulin-dependent diabetes mellitus
NNRTI	non-nucleoside reverse transcriptase inhibitor
NO	nitric oxide
NPO	nil per os (nothing by mouth)
NSAID	nonsteroidal anti-inflammatory drug
Nuc	nuclear medicine
NYHA	New York Heart Association
OB	obstetric
OCD	obsessive-compulsive disorder
OCPs	oral contraceptive pills
OR	operating room
PA	posteroanterior
PABA	para-aminobenzoic acid
PAN	polyarteritis nodosa
P-ANCA	perinuclear antineutrophil cytoplasmic antibody
Pa_{O_2}	partial pressure of oxygen in arterial blood
PAS	periodic acid Schiff
PAT	paroxysmal atrial tachycardia
PBS	peripheral blood smear
P_{CO_2}	partial pressure of carbon dioxide
PCOM	posterior communicating (artery)
PCOS	polycystic ovarian syndrome
PCP	phencyclidine
PCR	polymerase chain reaction
PCT	porphyria cutanea tarda
PCTA	percutaneous coronary transluminal angioplasty
PCV	polycythemia vera
PDA	patent ductus arteriosus
PDGF	platelet-derived growth factor
PE	physical exam
PEFR	peak expiratory flow rate
PEG	polyethylene glycol
PEPCK	phosphoenolpyruvate carboxykinase
PET	positron emission tomography
PFTs	pulmonary function tests
PID	pelvic inflammatory disease
PIP	proximal interphalangeal (joint)
PKU	phenylketonuria
PMDD	premenstrual dysphoric disorder
PML	progressive multifocal leukoencephalopathy
PMN	polymorphonuclear (leukocyte)
PNET	primitive neuroectodermal tumor
PNH	paroxysmal nocturnal hemoglobinuria
P_{O_2}	partial pressure of oxygen
PPD	purified protein derivative (of tuberculosis)
PPH	primary postpartum hemorrhage

PRA	panel reactive antibody
PROM	premature rupture of membranes
PSA	prostate-specific antigen
PSS	progressive systemic sclerosis
PT	prothrombin time
PTH	parathyroid hormone
PTSD	post-traumatic stress disorder
PTT	partial thromboplastin time
PUVA	psoralen ultraviolet A
PVC	premature ventricular contraction
RA	rheumatoid arthritis
RAIU	radioactive iodine uptake
RAST	radioallergosorbent test
RBC	red blood cell
REM	rapid eye movement
RES	reticuloendothelial system
RFFIT	rapid fluorescent focus inhibition test
RFTs	renal function tests
RHD	rheumatic heart disease
RNA	ribonucleic acid
RNP	ribonucleoprotein
RPR	rapid plasma reagin
RR	respiratory rate
RSV	respiratory syncytial virus
RUQ	right upper quadrant
RV	residual volume
Sao_2	oxygen saturation in arterial blood
SBFT	small bowel follow-through
SCC	squamous cell carcinoma
SCID	severe combined immunodeficiency
SERM	selective estrogen receptor modulator
SGOT	serum glutamic-oxaloacetic transaminase
SIADH	syndrome of inappropriate antidiuretic hormone
SIDS	sudden infant death syndrome
SLE	systemic lupus erythematosus
SMA	superior mesenteric artery
SSPE	subacute sclerosing panencephalitis
SSRI	selective serotonin reuptake inhibitor
ST	stable toxin
STD	sexually transmitted disease
T2W	T2-weighted (MRI)
T_3	triiodothyronine
T_4	thyroxine
TAH-BSO	total abdominal hysterectomy–bilateral salpingo-oophorectomy
TB	tuberculosis
TCA	tricyclic antidepressant

TCC	transitional cell carcinoma
TDT	terminal deoxytransferase
TFTs	thyroid function tests
TGF	transforming growth factor
THC	tetrahydrocannabinol
TIA	transient ischemic attack
TLC	total lung capacity
TMP-SMX	trimethoprim-sulfamethoxazole
tPA	tissue plasminogen activator
TP-HA	*Treponema pallidum* hemagglutination assay
TPP	thiamine pyrophosphate
TRAP	tartrate-resistant acid phosphatase
tRNA	transfer ribonucleic acid
TSH	thyroid-stimulating hormone
TSS	toxic shock syndrome
TTP	thrombotic thrombocytopenic purpura
TURP	transurethral resection of the prostate
TXA	thromboxane A
UA	urinalysis
UDCA	ursodeoxycholic acid
UGI	upper GI
UPPP	uvulopalatopharyngoplasty
URI	upper respiratory infection
US	ultrasound
UTI	urinary tract infection
UV	ultraviolet
VDRL	Venereal Disease Research Laboratory
VIN	vulvar intraepithelial neoplasia
VIP	vasoactive intestinal polypeptide
VLDL	very low density lipoprotein
VMA	vanillylmandelic acid
V/Q	ventilation/perfusion (ratio)
VRE	vancomycin-resistant enterococcus
VS	vital signs
VSD	ventricular septal defect
vWF	von Willebrand's factor
VZV	varicella-zoster virus
WAGR	Wilms' tumor, aniridia, genitourinary abnormalities, mental retardation (syndrome)
WBC	white blood cell
WHI	Women's Health Initiative
WPW	Wolff-Parkinson-White syndrome
XR	x-ray
ZN	Ziehl-Neelsen (stain)

CASE 1

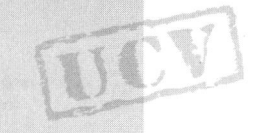

ID/CC A 30-year-old man who is known to have **full-blown AIDS** presents with **tremor, ataxia, memory loss, and both visual and auditory hallucinations.**

HPI He has no history of seizures, fever, neck stiffness, or vomiting.

PE No focal neurologic signs; fundus normal; no meningeal signs.

Labs LP: normal proteins in CSF; normal glucose. India ink staining negative (rule out cryptococcal meningitis); VDRL nonreactive (rule out neurosyphilis).

Imaging MR, brain: bright spots (on T2 weighted); cortical atrophy and ventricular dilatation.

Gross Pathology Diffuse leukoencephalopathy with enlargement of cortical sulci and ventricles.

Treatment Combination antiretroviral therapy may improve neuropsychiatric symptoms; no definitive treatment available.

Discussion AIDS dementia complex is characterized by a **progressive dementia, psychomotor abnormalities, focal motor abnormalities, and behavioral changes.** Clinical manifestations of this disorder are found in at least two-thirds of patients with AIDS. However, neurologic manifestations in the HIV-infected individual may be associated with CNS disease caused by such organisms as *Cryptococcus neoformans, Toxoplasma gondii, Treponema pallidum*, and JC virus (progressive multifocal leukoencephalopathy) as well as with B-cell lymphoma.

CASE 2

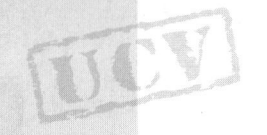

ID/CC An 18-year-old man in the postdrome of a 12-day admission due to herpes simplex encephalitis reports anxiety caused by an **inability to recall events that occurred just before his hospitalization.**

HPI He also reports tingling of the buttocks since his illness.

Discussion Amnestic disorder often occurs as a result of pathologic processes (e.g., closed head trauma, penetrating wounds, surgical intervention, hypoxia, infarction of the posterior cerebral artery and its distributions, and encephalitis) that cause damage to specific diencephalic and mediotemporal lobe structures, such as the mammillary bodies, fornices, and hippocampus. **Herpes simplex infection is the most common cause of viral encephalitis in teenagers and young adults.** Amnesia may be transient (less than 1 month in duration) or chronic.

CASE 3

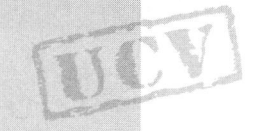

ID/CC A 14-year-old male is brought by his neighbor to the ER after being found in a **confused, hostile state** with a cut over his right eye.

HPI Further questioning of the neighbor reveals that the patient and his friend had been **inhaling turpentine** in the neighbor's garage. The boy was brought to the neighbor's attention after he exhibited strange behavior.

Treatment **Haloperidol**, a neuroleptic, or benzodiazepines should be given as sedating agents. Because the patient is under 18 years of age, child protective services should be contacted. The child's family should be informed about his actions and counseled.

CASE 4

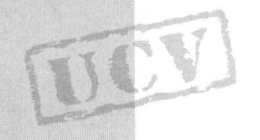

ID/CC A 72-year-old white woman hospitalized for 2 days with lobar pneumonia is restrained because of her **attempts to rise from bed** and pull out an IV line.

HPI She appears **confused and anxious** and responds to questions with **rambling, incoherent speech**. Before her hospitalization, she had been living on her own. Her daughter denies any recent change in her mother's ability to take care of herself and **denies any use of drugs or alcohol** by her mother.

PE VS: fever (39°C). PE: mini-mental status exams over past 2 days suggest **fluctuations in attention, orientation, and cognitive ability with generalized progressive degeneration**; consolidation in lower left lung with rales throughout.

Imaging CT, head: normal.

Treatment As many cues as possible should be supplied to allow patient to maintain a sense of time and place as well as a sense of security. If possible, a familiar family member or a 24-hour sitter should stay with patient at all times. A clock, calendar, or television may be used to orient patient to waking and sleeping hours. A neuroleptic agent (e.g., haloperidol) can be used if necessary to control agitation. Attempts should be made to eliminate underlying medical cause (e.g., infections or polypharmacy).

Discussion Delirium is especially common in the elderly.

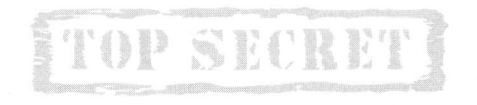

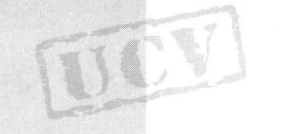

CASE 5

NEUROLOGY

ID/CC A 63-year-old male complains to his family physician of **progressive memory impairment**.

HPI The patient **cannot remember his home address**. His wife reports that he was forced to stop working because he was making an increasing number of mistakes. She also reports a few brief episodes during which he has appeared dazed and uncommunicative.

PE VS: BP normal. PE: no evidence of organic CNS pathology; **recent memory impairment on mental status exam** without impaired consciousness.

Imaging CT, head: diffuse atrophy and prominent sulci.

Micro Pathology **Neurofibrillary tangles** and **amyloid plaque** development are commonly seen in neurons of hippocampus.

Treatment No specific cure; supportive management; caregiver counseling; **acetylcholinesterase inhibitors (tacrine, donepezil)** and **vitamin E** may have some benefit.

Discussion Characterized by **degeneration of cholinergic neurons in the nucleus basalis**. The APP gene on chromosome 21 has been shown to be defective in a small subset of Alzheimer's patients. Alzheimer's disease is the most common cause of dementia in people over age 65.

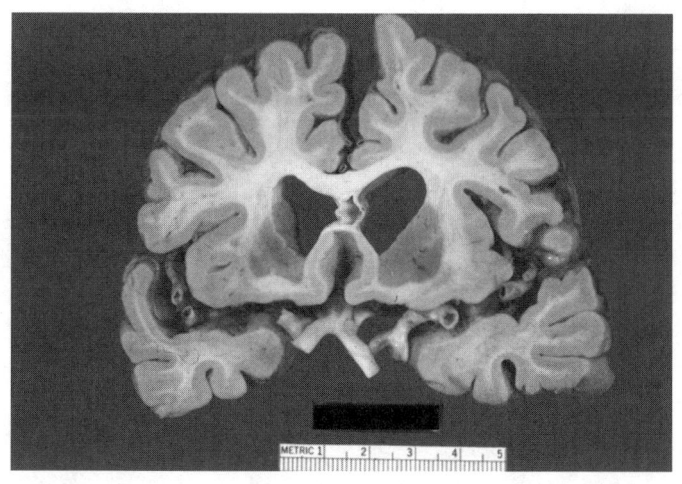

Figure 005 Diffuse cortical atrophy with mild enlargement of the lateral ventricles, widened sulci and narrowed gyri.

CASE 6

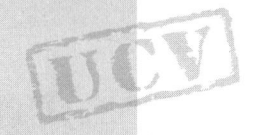

ID/CC A 67-year-old woman is brought to the ER by her daughter because of a **sudden** diminishment in cognitive ability and left-sided gait disturbance.

HPI Her daughter reports that the patient "was fine just this morning."

PE VS: irregular pulse; **hypertension**. PE: mini-mental status exam score 22/30; speech slurred; neurologic examination reveals left leg paresthesia, weakness of flexor and extensor muscles, and diminished reflexes.

Labs Normal motor conductance in muscles of left leg on EMG.

Imaging MR: multiple small **cerebral infarctions**.

Treatment Supportive treatment and rehabilitation; stroke prevention with antihypertensives, anticoagulants, and hypolipidemic agents as appropriate.

Discussion Patients with multi-infarct dementia exhibit **stepwise decline in mental function** (due to multiple small infarctions).

CASE 7

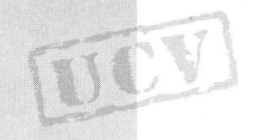

NEUROLOGY

ID/CC A 15-year-old white male presents with a 3-month history of **sudden, brief, irrepressible daytime sleep attacks, bilateral loss of muscle tone** (CATAPLEXY), and recurrent episodes of **REM sleep within minutes of falling asleep.**

HPI He sometimes has **dreamlike auditory or visual hallucinations** while falling asleep (HYPNAGOGIC) and awakening (HYPNOPOMPIC). Occasionally he finds himself **paralyzed** for a few seconds **while awakening**. He denies any drug use and is not on any medications.

PE Physical examination normal.

Labs Sleep apnea or loud snoring may be present; EEG shows that patient's sleep cycle begins with REM sleep.

Treatment **Methylphenidate**, a stimulant, may be used to prevent daytime sleep. **Imipramine** may be added if cataplexy is a significant component of the disorder. Benzodiazepines may be used to control insomnia, which can accompany presenting symptoms. Continuous positive airway pressure (CPAP) may be helpful in some cases if sleep apnea is involved.

Discussion Narcolepsy affects roughly 1 in every 2000 people and is associated with a strong genetic component. The differential includes myxedema, hypercapnia, brain tumor, Kleine-Levin syndrome (hyperphagia, hypersomnia, and hypersexuality), and Pickwickian syndrome (obesity with respiratory insufficiency). The **patient progresses from an awake and alert state of consciousness directly into REM sleep.** Sleep attacks last for about 5 minutes.

CASE 8

ID/CC A 10-year-old male "spaces out" during class and exhibits a slight quivering of his lips.

HPI These **brief seizures** happen several times a day, each lasting from a few seconds to a minute. The boy's teachers report that the child exhibits **no postictal confusion** but add that at times he **does not know that he has had a seizure**. He wears a helmet to prevent injury in the event of a seizure while walking.

Labs EEG: **3-Hz spikes and slow-wave activity**.

Imaging MR, brain: normal.

Treatment Pharmacologic therapy with **ethosuximide** and/or valproic acid.

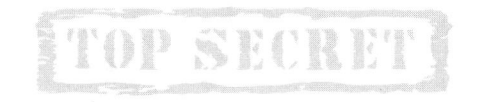

Discussion Seizures tend to occur in childhood and often resolve with age. They should be differentiated from conversion disorders and dissociative disorders.

CASE 9

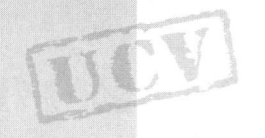

NEUROLOGY

ID/CC A 25-year-old male is brought to the ER in a **drowsy state**; according to his wife, he was working in the house when he **suddenly lost consciousness** and fell to the ground.

HPI His wife reports that after he lost consciousness, his **respiration temporarily ceased**. This episode lasted for about 45 seconds and was followed by **jerking of all four limbs** for about 3 to 4 minutes. The patient was then unconscious for an additional 3 to 4 minutes. He has no history of fever, neck stiffness, or vomiting.

PE VS: normal. PE: large laceration on lip; fundus normal; no meningeal signs; no focal neurologic deficit; vitals maintained.

Labs Lytes: normal. Blood glucose normal. EEG: **normal background interrupted by generalized spike and slow-wave discharges** ranging from 3 to 5 Hz; can be elicited by hyperventilation, photic stimulation, and sleep.

Imaging CT, head: normal.

Treatment Anticonvulsant therapy with phenytoin or valproate.

Discussion A seizure is a paroxysmal, abnormal discharge of neurons of the cerebral cortex that alters neurologic function. Epilepsy is a heterogeneous condition characterized by recurrent, unprovoked seizures. More than 10% of the population of the United States will have a seizure at some time during their lives, and epilepsy will develop in 1% to 2% of the population.

CASE 10

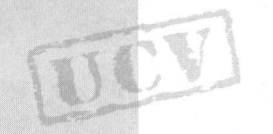

ID/CC A 40-year-old woman presents with a history of seizures characterized by an **aura of foul odor** at onset followed by **isolated jerking of the right thumb** and then the right hand, **spreading to the right arm** and then to the right side of the face without any loss of consciousness.

HPI She states that she has **never lost consciousness** during any of her seizures.

PE No focal neurologic deficit noted during interictal period.

Labs EEG: regularly occurring spike discharges in left motor cortex during interictal period.

Treatment **Carbamazepine** is drug of choice; newer agents such as gabapentin or lamotrigine may be useful.

Discussion Simple-partial seizures **begin locally in the brain and spread outward to adjacent cortical structures.** They can be motor, sensory, autonomic, or psychic and may secondarily generalize.

CASE 11

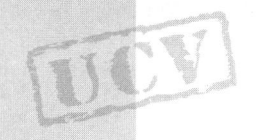

ID/CC A 35-year-old woman presents with a 14-month history of episodes in which she loses contact with her surroundings.

HPI The patient's first episode was brought to her attention by a friend, who noticed that she **suddenly got a vague look in her eyes and started smacking her lips** and rubbing her right thumb against her left hand for 20 to 60 seconds. In recent months, the patient has also noticed a **foul odor and taste in her mouth**.

PE No focal neurologic signs.

Labs EEG: left-sided spikes; **sharp wave discharges over frontotemporal regions** both interictally and during seizure.

Imaging PET: temporal lobe hypometabolism interictally.

Treatment Carbamazepine is drug of choice; newer agents such as gabapentin or lamotrigine may be useful.

Discussion Temporal lobe epilepsy can present with a **wide range of abnormal behaviors**, including labile affect, auditory hallucinations, and even paranoid ideation.

CASE 12

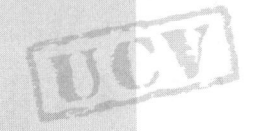

ID/CC A 33-year-old male arrives in the ER in **continuous seizure**.

HPI Upon regaining consciousness after a period of **postictal confusion**, he reports that he was **previously diagnosed with epilepsy** and recently **stopped taking his medication**.

PE Examination to rule out heart disease, meningitis, and increased intracranial pressure produces no findings; no papilledema; no nuchal rigidity on passive neck flexion.

Labs EEG: **typical epileptic spikes**. ECG: regular sinus rhythm. LP: normal opening pressure; slightly elevated protein.

Imaging CT, head: no intracranial bleeding or mass lesions.

Treatment Status epilepticus is a **medical emergency**; IV diazepam or lorazepam should be administered immediately. Prolonged status epilepticus can result in permanent brain damage. After the acute event has resolved, preventive pharmacologic therapy should be started. Carbamazepine, phenytoin, primidone, and phenobarbital have all been used with some success.

Discussion The differential diagnosis includes meningitis, brain abscess, stroke, head trauma, metabolic disturbances (e.g., hyponatremia), drug reaction, alcohol/anticonvulsant drug withdrawal, vitamin B_6 deficiency, and panic attack.

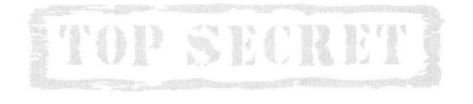

CASE 13

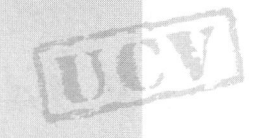

ID/CC — A 17-year-old male is brought to the ER by the police because of cold exposure; he had casually left his parents' home after **destroying furniture** and appliances in their living room **following an argument** they had had about his curfew.

HPI — Interview of his parents reveals that the young man is a **promising student** but has had disciplinary problems at school and at home. This episode marked **the most exaggerated and aggressive of his many outbursts**, although it is characterized by lack of emotion on his part.

PE — VS: tachycardia; skin cold and clammy (due to peripheral vasoconstriction).

Discussion — Acting out is an action-level **ego defense mechanism** in which the individual **deals with emotional conflict or internal or external stressors through actions rather than reflections or feelings**. Acting out should be differentiated from other inappropriate behavior on the basis of evidence relating behavior to emotional conflict.

CASE 14

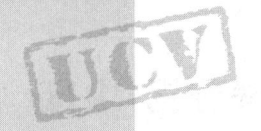

ID/CC A 35-year-old male is diagnosed with ischemic heart disease following an evaluation for an episode of anginal chest pain; on the following day he is **found doing push-ups prior to a medical consultation.**

HPI On further interview, he states that there is **"nothing wrong" with him** and that "it's all just an overreaction."

Discussion The defense mechanism employed here is denial. The patient finds it difficult to believe he is ill and uses **denial to cope** with the difficult news of his illness.

CASE 15

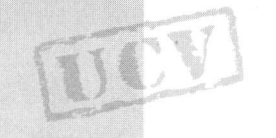

ID/CC A 34-year-old woman presenting for her annual gynecologic exam erupts into tears upon hearing that her Pap smear showed atypical cells, announcing between sobs that "things like this always happen" to her.

HPI She rejects attempts to comfort her, stating that "that's the way things are; stupid things happen to useless people." She continues by calling herself a whore and states that the finding is an appropriate punishment for the sexual promiscuity of her youth.

Discussion Devaluation is an image-distorting ego defense mechanism in which an individual deals with emotional conflict or internal or external stressors by attributing exaggerated negative qualities to self.

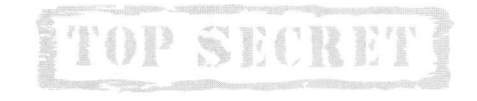

CASE 16

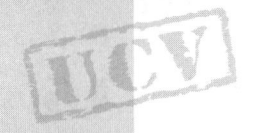

ID/CC   A physician seeing her first patient of the day is **uncharacteristically forceful** in advising that patient to lose weight.

HPI   She had an **argument with her son** the previous night, during which he again refused to take what she considered to be sound advice.

Discussion   The defense mechanism being used by the physician is displacement. Displacement involves the **transfer of emotions** from an **unacceptable to an acceptable person or object** and has been associated with the development of phobias in psychodynamic theory.

CASE 17

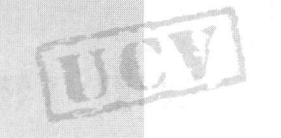

ID/CC — A 27-year-old male professional presents to the internist for a work physical; the visit proceeds normally until the subject of his sexual history arises, at which time the patient becomes **overtly shy**, no longer looks directly at the examiner, and begins to **giggle**.

HPI — Further inquiry about past sexual activity only enhances his shy behavior. **Normal mature behavior returns** with continuation of the remaining history.

PE — Physical exam normal; patient again demonstrates shy and embarrassed behavior during the urogenital exam.

Discussion — Fixation is an ego defense mechanism marked by a partial or localized **paralysis at a more childish level of development**.

DEFENSE MECHANISM

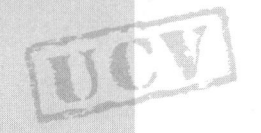

CASE 18

ID/CC	A 37-year-old woman presents with lower abdominal pain, lethargy, and pain on defecation.
HPI	Questioning reveals that the patient's **symptoms began soon after her spouse's death** from colon cancer.
PE	Abdomen tender to palpation.
Labs	Stool guaiac negative.
Imaging	Colonoscopy reveals no abnormalities.
Treatment	Psychotherapy may be beneficial.
Discussion	Identification is an **ego defense mechanism** in which a person's **behavior is unconsciously patterned after someone else**; it is often associated with **child abuse or loss**.

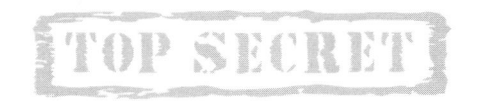

CASE 19

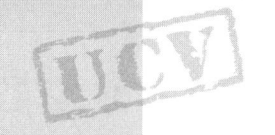

ID/CC A 24-year-old medical student recounts his experience in gross anatomy to his family over the Thanksgiving holiday.

HPI His **emotionless and scientific narrative** is interrupted by his sister's surprise that he has **not harbored any of the concern and guilt** that he had expected to encounter in the process of dissection.

Discussion Isolation of affect is an **inhibitory ego defense mechanism** characterized by a **separation of feelings from ideas and events**.

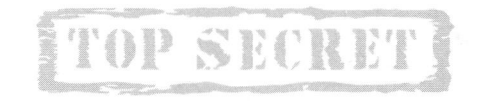

CASE 20

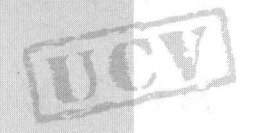

ID/CC — A 28-year-old man presents for an annual physical; after testing positive for gonorrhea, he reveals that he has been cheating on his wife, stating that **she cares more about her career than she cares about him**.

HPI — He loves his wife and feels compatible with her, but while she was struggling to earn a promotion, he engaged in numerous affairs.

Treatment — Psychotherapy can help by bringing true issues out so that they can be discussed.

Discussion — Rationalization is a **subconscious process** in which a person **relieves some of his or her anxieties** about doing something socially unacceptable **by providing a logical reason for doing it**.

CASE 21

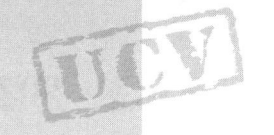

ID/CC A 15-year-old boy being seen for a sports physical reveals his disgust at his best friend's confession that he might be gay, stating that he "can't stand being near that faggot" and that "all homosexuals should go to hell."

HPI He and the young man have been best friends for years; he admits that he has never been closer to anyone else. He appears shaken by the process of recounting his experience.

Discussion Reaction formation is an **inhibitory ego defense mechanism** marked by the **replacement of a personally unacceptable idea or feeling by an emphasis on its opposite**. In this case, the patient has structured a strong homophobia to deny any possibility of attraction to his male friend.

DEFENSE MECHANISM

CASE 22

ID/CC A 24-year-old woman with a history of systemic lupus erythematosus (SLE) **begins bedwetting** and **throwing tantrums** at her biweekly appointments for dialysis.

HPI Since being diagnosed with SLE, she has had to leave graduate school and **move in with her parents**. She has found dialysis to be a painful and very trying experience and often **sucks her thumb** to ease her anxiety.

Discussion Regression is characterized by **childlike behavior under stress**, such as physical illness or hospitalization.

CASE 23

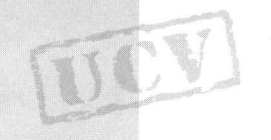

ID/CC A witness of an appalling crime visits his physician because he **cannot recall** any details about the assailant.

HPI Despite the patient's repeated efforts, he cannot elicit this memory.

Treatment Hypnosis has proven useful in some cases.

Discussion **Repression is the involuntary exclusion of painful memories** or impulses from awareness. **Suppression is the exclusion of painful memories or impulses resulting from conscious effort** (e.g., to stop thinking about an upsetting event without actually forgetting that event).

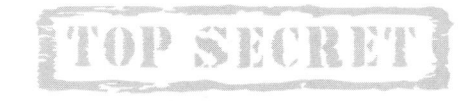

DEFENSE MECHANISM

CASE 24

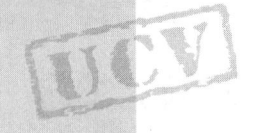

ID/CC A patient who has been hospitalized for coronary bypass surgery describes the house staff as either **angelic or demonic**.

HPI Further questioning reveals that this **dichotomy** also encompasses the patient's understanding of his **relationship to his family and to people at work**.

Discussion Splitting involves a **compartmentalization of opposite affect states to deal with emotional conflict or internal or external stressors**. Because ambivalent affects cannot be experienced simultaneously, the patient's emotional awareness rests on an exclusion of balanced views and expectations of self and others. **Often seen in patients with personality disorders, especially borderline personality**.

CASE 25

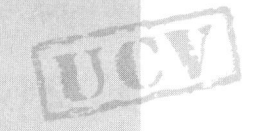

ID/CC A 27-year-old man tells his physician of his decision to go into civic law upon his graduation from law school this summer.

HPI He plans to pursue a career in criminal prosecution law despite his father's desire that he enter a more lucrative field. He repeatedly mentions that his brother was killed by a drunk driver who received a minimal sentence.

Discussion In sublimation, an **unacceptable instinctual impulse is channeled into a socially acceptable action**. Here, the unacceptable desire for vengeance through vigilantism was channeled into a desire to become a criminal prosecutor. Considered a "mature" defense mechanism.

CASE 26

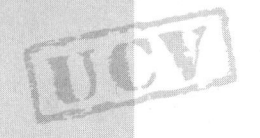

ID/CC A 28-year-old woman presents with a 3-month history of **anxiety and depression following her breakup with her fiancé** of 3 years.

HPI She has been **overwhelmed by feelings of sadness, tearfulness, and depression** and is concerned that she will never be in a relationship again or fulfill her dream of having a family. Since her breakup with her fiancé, she has **lost touch with friends and family**, and her **performance at work has steadily declined**.

PE Physical exam reveals a cachectic and poorly groomed woman.

Discussion Adjustment disorder (AD) is characterized by the **development of clinically significant emotional or behavioral symptoms in response to an identifiable psychosocial stressor or stressors**. The symptoms must develop within 3 months after the onset of the stressor. ADs are coded according to the subtype that best characterizes the predominant symptoms. In this case, the patient would be diagnosed as adjustment disorder with mixed anxiety and depressed mood.

CASE 27

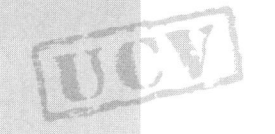

ID/CC A female patient complains of **uncontrollable anxiety of more than 6 months' duration** together with daily symptoms that she attributes to a heart condition.

HPI The symptoms interfere with her social and professional life because she never knows when the anxiety will begin. She is **irritable, fatigues easily, has poor concentration**, and has **difficulty falling asleep**. She reports that during the exacerbations, her heart beats quickly, she sweats, and she occasionally has diarrhea. The patient has no specific phobias.

Labs Normal cardiac enzymes. ECG: regular sinus rhythm. Normal TSH level.

Treatment Buspirone; some patients may benefit from short-term low-dose benzodiazepines; antidepressants may also confer benefit, particularly selective serotonin reuptake inhibitors (SSRIs). Patients should be counseled to maintain a productive lifestyle. Acute anxiety can be managed with biofeedback and meditation. Heart palpitations may be controlled with beta-blockers.

Discussion In roughly half of all patients, the disorder resolves with time. Before diagnosing generalized anxiety disorder, **rule out thyroid disorders and pheochromocytoma**.

CASE 28

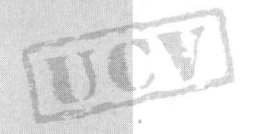

ID/CC A 21-year-old female student having a routine physical exam appears distracted and focused on the office ceiling; when confronted by the physician, she is embarrassed but admits that she is **counting the number of tiles on the ceiling.**

HPI For the past 5 months, she has experienced an **irresistible urge to count objects** on a daily basis. She estimates that she spends 1 to 2 hours counting tiles each morning, often **missing her classes or meetings** as a result. The patient adds that she is **distressed by the unreasonable amount of time** she spends on such activities but feels that she can't stop. She denies any substance abuse or use of medications.

Labs Lab work normal.

Treatment **Exposure therapy** and other types of **behavioral therapy** have been proven useful. Obsessive-compulsive disorder (OCD) may involve dysfunction of cortical **serotonin** systems. **Clomipramine**, a tricyclic antidepressant, has been shown to have an effect on OCD symptoms. **Selective serotonin reuptake inhibitors (SSRIs)** are also useful.

Discussion The prevalence of obsessive-compulsive disorder is estimated to be 1%. Onset occurs most often in adolescence or early adulthood. This disorder can manifest itself in the form of **compulsive habits** or **persistent thoughts or images** that are perceived as **intrusive** (obsessions) and that cause the patient significant distress.

CASE 29

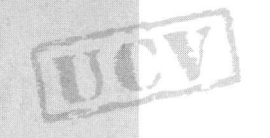

ID/CC A 57-year-old man is brought to the ER following an episode of **chest pain, dizziness, diaphoresis, and shortness of breath** which ended in syncope.

HPI He is somewhat confused by his arrival at the hospital. Workup reveals **no signs of MI**. Further questioning reveals that the patient has had **numerous such episodes** in the past, each preceded by **thoughts of speaking before the executive board** of his company.

Labs ECG: no ST depression or elevation; no other evidence of myocardial damage.

Treatment Benzodiazepines to alleviate acute symptoms. Behavioral therapy (systematic desensitization and cognitive therapy) has shown success in enabling the individual to counteract anxiety brought about by panic triggers.

Discussion Panic disorder is **characterized by discrete periods of intense fear or discomfort** peaking in 10 minutes with four of the following: (1) palpitations and racing heart; (2) sweating; (3) trembling; (4) shortness of breath; (5) choking feeling; (6) chest pain; (7) nausea/abdominal distress; (8) dizziness, faintness, and lightheadedness; (9) derealization; (10) fear of losing control; (11) fear of dying; (12) paresthesias; and (13) chills or hot flashes. Panic disorder must be diagnosed in a certain context, e.g., panic disorder with agoraphobia. In this case, the patient's panic attack was elicited by his fear of public speaking.

ANXIETY DISORDERS

CASE 30

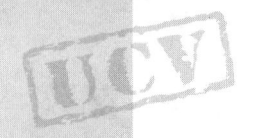

ID/CC — A war veteran complains of **intense and vivid flashbacks** with associated **anxiety and hyperarousal**.

HPI — The patient has **witnessed and experienced traumatic events** but **cannot recall** certain details of these events, and he **becomes anxious** both when questioned about the events and **when he encounters cues that remind him of them**. He also reports **difficulty falling asleep, hypervigilance**, emotional outbursts, difficulty concentrating, and recurrent nightmares that have begun to **interfere with his life**.

PE — Patient appears anxious.

Treatment — Counseling should begin as soon after the traumatic event as possible. Some patients may benefit from benzodiazepines (for anxiety) and antidepressants.

Discussion — Seventy-five percent of patients drop out of counseling programs because remembering the traumatic event is too anxiety-provoking. PTSD may be classified as **acute (duration of 3 months or less)** or **chronic (duration of more than 3 months)**.

CASE 31

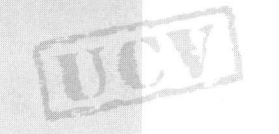

ID/CC A 36-year-old woman tells her physician that **she turned down a promotion at work** because her new duties would have included **speaking in front of the company's executive board.**

HPI She is upset about her decision but maintains that she "**just couldn't get up in front of them.**"

Treatment **Cognitive behavioral psychotherapy** is the most effective treatment; MAO inhibitors and selective serotonin reuptake inhibitors (SSRIs) may be helpful for generalized social phobia. Beta-blockers or benzodiazepines may alleviate anxiety on an as-needed basis in specific social phobias (e.g., test-taking or performance anxiety).

Discussion Exposure to the feared situation almost invariably causes anxiety in patients with social phobia. The individual recognizes that the fear is an unreasonable one. Frequent comorbidity with substance abuse and depression.

CASE 32

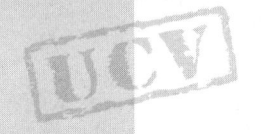

ID/CC — An 8-year-old male is brought to the family physician by his mother because he makes careless mistakes, **cannot maintain his concentration or listen to commands**, and is forgetful, hyperactive, and noisy.

HPI — He has been like this for **at least 6 months**. He also shows **poor impulse control**. His performance in school has suffered, and he has few friends. There is no history of psychosis.

PE — Patient appears restless and **fidgets continuously**; physical and mental development normal for age.

Treatment — **Treatment of choice** is a **stimulant**, most commonly methylphenidate (Ritalin), and supportive family therapy.

Discussion — There are three types of ADHD: **attention-deficit predominant type**, formerly known as attention deficit disorder (ADD); **hyperactivity predominant type**; and **combined type**. Children with ADHD are often placed in classes for those with learning disabilities because they are unable to concentrate.

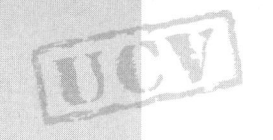

CASE 33

ID/CC — A 4-year-old boy presents with **severe language delay** together with an **inability to interact with other children or adults**; his parents say that he spends a great deal of time **spinning around in circles**.

HPI — His parents state that they noticed nothing unusual in infancy except the child's **indifference to being cuddled**.

PE — Physical development normal; intelligence subnormal; child is **not interactive** and exhibits **repetitive behavior**.

Labs — Serum serotonin level elevated; other tests normal.

Treatment — Aim therapy at increasing social and communication skills and at improving self-care ability. Group therapy with autistic or normal peers may yield improved social function.

Discussion — Autistic disorder is a **pervasive developmental disorder** that begins before three years of age and is found in 0.05% of all children. Of these, only 2% can live independently; most remain severely impaired throughout their lives. Children with pure mental retardation can be distinguished from those with infantile autism in that they do not exhibit bizarre behavior or deficits in social relations.

CASE 34

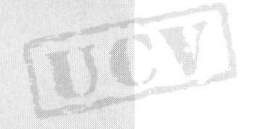

ID/CC A 10-month-old female is brought to the doctor by her mother, who feels that the baby is retarded, cannot see properly, and falls repeatedly; the child has **bruises in different stages of healing** (suggestive of child abuse).

PE No lacerations or fractures noted; normal physical development for 10 months of age; **bilateral retinal hemorrhages** seen; skin, sclera, joints normal.

Labs Coagulation profile normal.

Imaging XR: no old or new fractures seen.

Treatment **Health care workers are required by law to report any suspicion of child abuse or neglect to state protection agencies**; victims are immediately removed from homes and placed in protective custody of a hospital or state facility.

Discussion Vigorous shaking can produce **vitreous and retinal hemorrhages** that may be the only verifiable signs of child abuse.

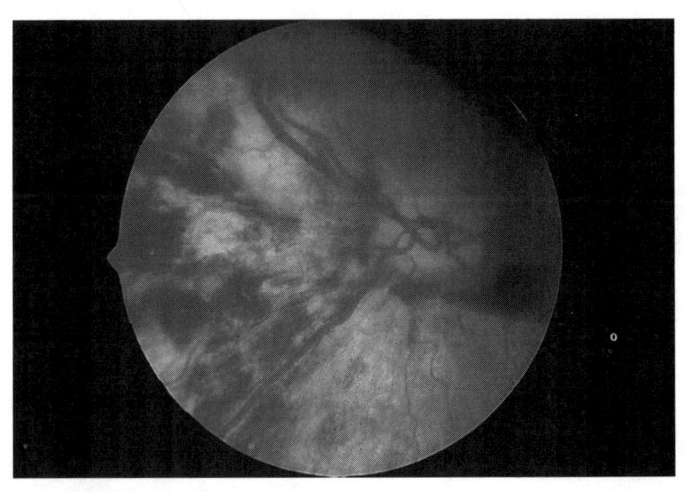

Figure 034 Diffuse microvascular hemorrhages.

CASE 35

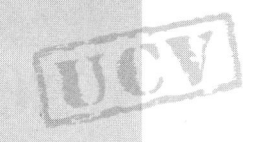

ID/CC A 10-year-old schoolboy is brought in for a consultation because he **fails to follow school rules** and shows **no concern for the feelings of others**.

HPI He has been known to trick his fellow students into giving him their lunch money. His teacher feels that he suffers from a behavioral disorder and needs psychiatric treatment.

PE Physical exam normal; physical and mental development normal for age.

Labs Routine tests within normal range.

Treatment Behavioral therapy.

Discussion Conduct disorder involves **failure to follow social norms** and corresponds to an **increased risk of criminal behavior in adults**. Associated with antisocial personality disorder in adulthood.

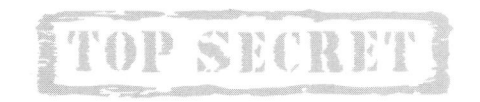

CHILD PSYCHIATRY

CASE 36

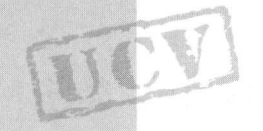

ID/CC A 6-year-old boy is brought by his mother to the family physician because of a 7-month history of episodic bedwetting.

HPI The child is **ashamed** to talk about his experience. His mother reports that his **performance in school has markedly decreased** in the past months. He has no history of seizures or spina bifida.

Labs Fasting blood glucose level normal (rule out juvenile diabetes).

Treatment Therapy should be directed toward both the problem itself and its psychological consequences.

Discussion Enuresis is defined as **urinary incontinence that is not due to a medical condition**. It may be voluntary or involuntary and can occur during the day or, more commonly, at night. Differential diagnosis should include neurogenic bladder, medical conditions that cause polyuria or urgency (e.g., juvenile diabetes, spina bifida, seizure disorder), and acute UTI. **Most children with the disorder become continent by adolescence.**

CASE 37

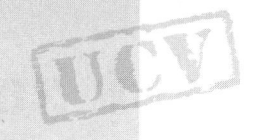

ID/CC A 4-year-old girl is brought to the physician by her drug-abusing mother for an evaluation of **developmental delay**, repetitive play, and **underdeveloped language skills**.

HPI Although the patient's mother abstained from drug and alcohol use during pregnancy, her mother and father frequently became drunk and fought with each other after the child was born. Often the patient was caught in the middle. The mother reports that the patient frequently comes to her in the middle of the night complaining **of bad dreams**. The mother has also noted **repetitive destructive behavior**. The patient often locks her doll in the closet and, upon hearing sirens, runs around tearfully and screams. She is **hypervigilant** with strangers and is **easily startled**.

Treatment The most important aspect of treatment is ensuring safe home environment. Psychotherapy and tutoring are also beneficial.

Discussion Adults with PTSD can often describe clear flashbacks. Children, however, generally lack the ability to understand and communicate their experiences as clearly, and diagnosis must therefore be based on history and play observation. **Disorganized or agitated behavior**, **repetitive play**, or **frightening dreams** may be observed.

CHILD PSYCHIATRY

CASE 38

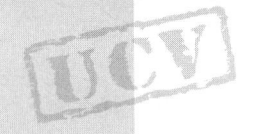

ID/CC A 5-year-old child develops **abdominal pain every Monday morning**.

HPI The child does not report any abnormality in his stools, and his parents have not noted any irregularity in his eating habits.

Labs Routine hemogram and stool exam fail to detect any abnormality.

Treatment Mild school avoidance should be managed with encouragement and by sending the child to school unless symptoms of illness are found. In more severe cases, a psychiatric referral should be made.

Discussion A child with separation anxiety may develop **functional symptoms** on days when he has to go to school; he feigns illness because it will keep him at home. Genetic factors, learning disabilities, mental retardation, and developmental immaturity may contribute to separation anxiety.

CASE 39

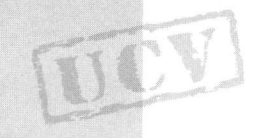

ID/CC A 47-year-old patient is referred by her family physician to a psychiatrist because her husband is concerned about a series of recent episodes in which the patient has **awoken screaming or crying** in the middle of the night.

HPI Her husband's attempts to awaken and comfort her are fruitless, and she gradually returns to peaceful sleep and **remembers nothing the next morning**. The episodes have been occurring every 3 to 4 days; however, they occurred every night while the patient's daughter was hospitalized for pneumonia.

Treatment Stress reduction measures and psychiatric evaluation.

Discussion Most patients do not awaken fully and have **amnesia for the episode in the morning**. Patients who do not experience amnesia for sleep terrors report fragmented fearful images rather than a storylike sequence (observed in nightmares). Sleep terrors **occur in delta sleep**, and patients exhibit intense fear and **autonomic arousal. Episode frequency increases with stress**.

CASE 40

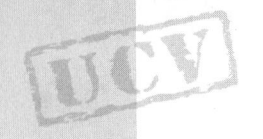

ID/CC An 8-year-old **male** is brought to his pediatrician with complaints of **repeated eye blinking, head jerking, and shoulder shrugging** of 2 years' duration.

HPI The patient has never had a tic-free period for more than 1 month. Recently, he has started making **involuntary sounds** that begin as slight grunts but progress to **loud barks and obscenities**.

PE Involuntary tics.

Treatment **Haloperidol** is effective in controlling tics. Psychotherapy may relieve stressful situations that may serve as precipitating factors.

Discussion **Dysfunctional regulation of dopamine** is most commonly involved in Gilles de la Tourette syndrome. It affects males three times more often than females; onset is most common before age 21.

CASE 41

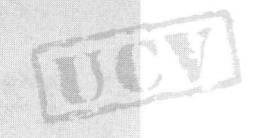

ID/CC A 17-year-old woman presents with amnesia over a 3-hour period following the death of a close friend.

HPI She reports no memory loss other than that concerning the period mentioned. She remembers in detail the last conversation she had with her friend but is **distressed** that she is unable to recall when her mother informed her of her friend's death. She **denies any substance abuse** or **recent physical trauma**.

Treatment Hospitalization may be helpful to remove threatening stimulus; psychotherapy to examine loss of memory. Psychotherapy is often very successful.

Discussion Dissociative amnesia is most common in adolescent and young adult females and is rare in the elderly. **Amnesia is localized and often follows a psychologically traumatic event.**

DISSOCIATIVE IDENTITY DISORDER

CASE 42

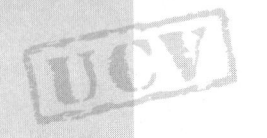

ID/CC A 24-year-old man presents with a history of **repeated episodes of anxiety-provoking detachment** during which he feels as if he is an external observer of his actions and thoughts.

HPI These episodes have occurred intermittently over the past 14 months. He also reports having felt **depressed** for long periods of time throughout the past year.

Treatment Pharmacologic interventions may be used for accompanying symptoms of anxiety, depression, or obsessions. Psychotherapy may be of value.

Discussion Depersonalization can occur in a number of disorders, including posttraumatic stress disorder (PTSD), substance abuse, and seizure disorders. Dissociative disorder is diagnosed with **recurrent episodes in the absence of these other disorders**.

CASE 43

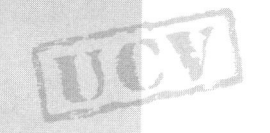

ID/CC — A 50-year-old woman who has lived in California all her life discovers that she is in Texas and does not know how she got there.

HPI — Her husband died in an automobile accident 2 weeks ago.

Treatment — Supportive psychotherapy.

Discussion — Dissociative fugue and dissociative amnesia both involve **failure to remember important information about oneself**. Dissociative fugue is further characterized by sudden, unexpected travel away from home with confusion about personal identity or even assumption of a new identity.

DISSOCIATIVE IDENTITY DISORDER

CASE 44

ID/CC — A 22-year-old woman presents to the emergency room in acute distress with a **2-hour history of amnesia** followed by what she describes as "**voices in her head**" telling her to kill herself.

HPI — She reports that these **amnesic episodes** have occurred before. She has tried to kill herself on two previous occasions, each time persuaded by the same voice that prompted her visit to the ER. She **denies any substance abuse** but has a **history of severe physical and emotional abuse as a child**.

PE — Sodium amylbarbital interview reveals second personality characterized by anger and disdain for patient's presenting personality; further questioning reveals that this personality has taken an active role in each of patient's suicide attempts.

Labs — **Shifts in personality correspond to changes in galvanic skin conductance, heart rate, muscle tone, visual acuity, and EEG wave patterns.**

Treatment — Psychotherapy and hypnotherapy should accompany medical therapy of associated disorders such as severe depression (selective serotonin reuptake inhibitors, tricyclics), psychoses (neuroleptics), and anxiety (benzodiazepines).

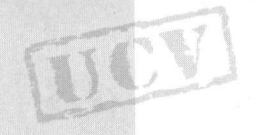

Discussion — Dissociative identity disorder was formerly referred to as **multiple personality disorder**.

CASE 45

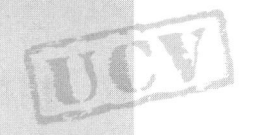

EATING DISORDERS

ID/CC A 14-year-old female is brought to the physician by her mother because her **body weight is less than 85% of that expected** and she has **missed her last three periods** (AMENORRHEA).

HPI The patient reports that she is fat and strongly fears gaining weight. She also reports intense hunger but prefers not to eat. She admits to abusing laxatives.

PE Patient severely underweight.

Labs Pregnancy test negative.

Treatment Individual and family therapy along with antidepressant medication; in severe cases, hospitalization may be required.

Discussion There are two major types of eating disorders: anorexia nervosa and bulimia. The current case describes anorexia nervosa. Females are 10 times more likely to be affected than males, and there is a higher incidence among those of upper to middle socioeconomic status. Anorexia nervosa has a 5% to 10% mortality rate.

CASE 46

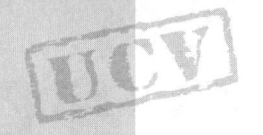

ID/CC A **20-year-old female college student** reveals a secret problem to her family physician.

HPI She has always been preoccupied by her body. **Several times a week**, she suffers **uncontrollable eating binges**. She almost always follows these binges with a visit to the bathroom, where she discreetly **makes herself vomit**. Following each such episode, **she feels depressed**.

Treatment Pharmacologic approach uses antidepressants; psychological approach uses psychotherapy, cognitive behavioral therapy.

Discussion Bulimia nervosa is characterized by **binge eating followed by purging**, which is accomplished by self-induced vomiting, laxative use, or use of diuretics. The prevalence of this condition in the United States is approximately 1.5% among young women but is rarely seen in men. The typical patient is usually somewhat underweight and binges and purges several times a week. Dietary intake may be very restricted, with nonpurged caloric intake averaging 1,000 kcal/day. Depression is often comorbid.

CASE 47

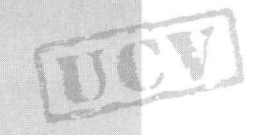

ID/CC A 37-year-old man presents for a work physical **to document loss of vision** that arose after **exposure to a volatile toxin at the work site.**

HPI There is no significant medical history. He reports total intractable blindness since the accident at work and is **seeking disability payments** from the company he works for.

PE VS: normal. PE: visual field testing demonstrates apparent total visual loss. Pupils equal, round, and reactive to light and accommodation; patient's eyes move rapidly back and forth when asked to fixate on numbers of a tape measure while the tape is being rapidly pulled out (OPTOKINETIC NYSTAGMUS; verifies that patient is feigning blindness).

Discussion Malingering is defined as **feigning illness or disability to escape work, elicit sympathy, or gain compensation.**

FACTITIOUS DISORDERS

CASE 48

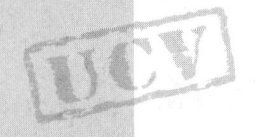

ID/CC A 37-year-old female with a history of insulin-dependent diabetes mellitus (IDDM) is admitted to the hospital for severe diabetic ketoacidosis (DKA).

HPI The patient is educated, articulate, and assertive and seems to be **extremely knowledgeable about her disease**. She claims that she controls her diabetes rigorously. After some phone inquiries, it is discovered that she has been admitted for hypoglycemia or DKA **at various local hospitals 23 times over the past 18 months**. When confronted with this finding, the patient becomes **angry and defensive** and leaves the hospital.

Labs Hyperglycemia (614 upon admission); HbA-1C 8% (elevation demonstrates poor long-term control of blood glucose).

Treatment It is important to **build rapport** when possible. The primary physician may want to interact with the patient in a **nonconfrontational** manner. Psychotherapy (with an emphasis on understanding etiology) may help, but the **prognosis is poor**.

Discussion Also known as **factitious disorder**, Munchausen's syndrome stems from a **conscious production of signs and symptoms of disease**. In this case, the patient's noncompliance was intentional. The aim of such patients is to **assume the sick role** when there is **no apparent benefit** to doing so.

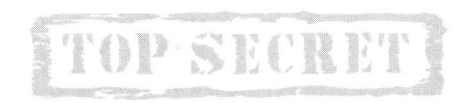

CASE 49

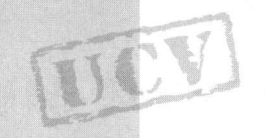

ID/CC A 10-year-old boy is brought to his family physician by his parents, who are concerned about his "feminine tendencies"; the boy's parents state that he continually **asks for clothes** and toys that are **designed for girls**, has **only female friends**, and on several occasions has been found **wearing his older sister's clothes**.

HPI The boy's parents claim that their son has always seemed to identify with the female gender. As a toddler, he protested at the prospect of being dressed in a suit and always sat while urinating. **The boy claims that he wants to be a girl** and adds that his favorite pastimes are games such as "house," in which he likes to **play "the wife."** His parents had hoped that he would grow out of this "phase" and are becoming increasingly concerned.

PE Physical exam unremarkable; normal male genitalia.

Treatment Adult patients may elect to undergo pharmacologic (e.g., estrogen) therapy or sex-reassignment surgery.

Discussion Gender identity disorder can be defined as a **persistent and powerful identification with the opposite gender**. It cannot stem from perceived social advantages associated with the other gender. Cross-gender behaviors tend not to continue into late adolescence. About three-fourths of such people subsequently report a bisexual or homosexual orientation. When gender identity continues into or begins in adulthood, it usually assumes a chronic course.

GENDER IDENTITY DISORDER

CASE 50

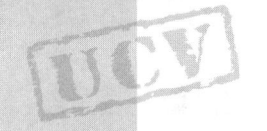

ID/CC A 40-year-old white female comes to the emergency room claiming that she is Jesus Christ.

HPI She is now medically stable and admits that she is not Jesus as "the voices" had told her. Over the past week, she has **slept fewer than 3 hours per night**. She initially excelled at work but recently became irritable and unable to concentrate. She then experienced **auditory command hallucinations** which told her that she had special powers. She recalls a similar episode several years ago and reports that occasionally she has felt depressed. She denies any drug use.

PE **Concentration impaired**; patient has flight of ideas; **speech rapid**; dressed in brightly colored clothes.

Labs TSH normal.

Treatment **Lithium** has been the traditional treatment of choice. Depakote and Tegretol are also effective treatments. Benzodiazepines and typical antipsychotic drugs may be useful short-term adjuncts.

Discussion More than 90% of bipolar disorder patients have a depressive episode. Manic episodes progress over days, and 20% of patients will have psychotic symptoms (**hallucinations and delusions**). Women are four times more likely than men to be rapid cyclers (i.e., to have four or more manic and depressive cycles per year).

CASE 51

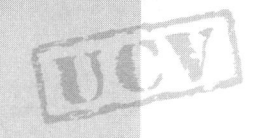

ID/CC — A 28-year-old male writer being seen for a routine annual physical reports recent **irritability and insomnia**.

HPI — He states that he has been extremely productive lately and that his work has demonstrated the value of his enhanced alertness. Upon further questioning, he reveals that he experiences these **hyperenergetic states episodically**; they are often **followed by periods of malaise, apathy, loss of appetite, decreased ability to concentrate, and hypersomnia** (MAJOR DEPRESSIVE EPISODE). He has considered these fluctuations to be a normal consequence of his work.

PE — Physical exam reveals a hyperalert but otherwise normal-appearing man.

Discussion — Bipolar II disorder should be considered in any case in which **hypomanic disorder is accompanied by prodrome or postdrome depression** that meets the criteria for major depressive disorder. Hypomanic disorder is similar to a manic episode except that mood disturbances are not severe enough to cause marked impairment in social or occupational functioning.

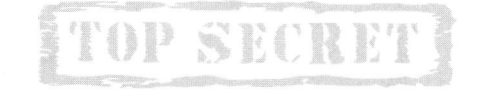

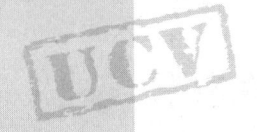

CASE 52

ID/CC A 16-year-old girl is brought by her mother to her family physician because of **mood fluctuations and poor performance** in school for the past year.

HPI She reports week-long **episodes of tiredness and generalized unhappiness over several years** (DYSTHYMIA) followed by **short periods of high energy and euphoria**. Her older brother is receiving treatment for depression.

Discussion Cyclothymic disorder entails a **2-year history** (1 year in children and adolescents) of numerous periods of **hypomanic symptoms** preceded or followed by **periods marked by depressive symptoms** that do not meet the criteria for a major depressive episode. There is a 15% to 50% risk that the person will subsequently develop bipolar I or II disorder.

CASE 53

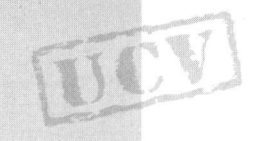

ID/CC An 80-year-old female who was recently diagnosed with breast cancer complains of **significant weight loss** and **forgetfulness** as well as multiple vague somatic complaints.

HPI She was scheduled for a mastectomy, and she had been undergoing presurgical evaluation. Her best friend died a few days ago.

PE Old, frail woman with hard lump in left breast; lymphadenopathy; no meningeal or focal neurologic signs; higher mental functions normal; no organomegaly found on abdominal exam; **admits to being depressed but denies any suicidal ideation**.

Treatment Antidepressant medication, psychiatric consultation. Watch for side effects of antidepressants in the elderly (orthostatic hypotension with tricyclic antidepressants).

Discussion The patient's recent and significant weight loss and her forgetfulness suggest that she is suffering from a major depressive episode. **Depression in the elderly often resembles pseudodementia** and can be treated effectively with antidepressant medication or electroconvulsive therapy.

CASE 54

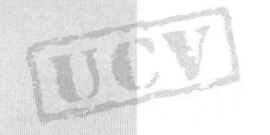

ID/CC A 42-year-old woman is brought by the police to the ER following a failed suicide attempt.

HPI The patient reports that she has felt **progressively sad** (DYSPHORIC) and **lacking in energy** over the past few months and has had **difficulty sleeping** over the same time period. She has **considered killing herself** numerous times but has only recently conceived of a plan by which to do so. She was recently fired because of her lethargy at work and has **lost interest in her long-time hobby** of reading. She feels **helpless** and **hopeless** about the state of her life and sees no solution other than to end it.

PE Depressed mood; restricted affect; suicidal ideation.

Treatment Assessment of suicide risk should be conducted before the patient is allowed to return home. Psychotherapy should accompany pharmacologic approaches to treatment of depression. Selective serotonin reuptake inhibitors (SSRIs) are considered first-line agents. Tricyclic agents and MAO inhibitors are considered second-line agents. Electroconvulsive therapy (ECT) is a consideration in recalcitrant and severe depression or if psychotic symptoms are present.

Discussion Suicide attempt rates in major depression have been found to be between 15% and 30%. Providers should be aware that asking questions about suicide ideation does not increase the chance that suicide will occur.

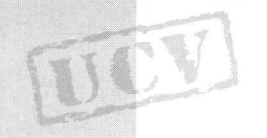

CASE 55

ID/CC A 50-year-old **female** attorney with a promising practice, two daughters, and a stable marriage is brought to her family physician for evaluation because her husband notes that she has "not been functioning properly" for the past 2 months.

HPI She has called her office frequently to tell her colleagues that she is ill, whereas in fact she was **unable to get out of bed in the morning**. She has **ceased to take pride in her appearance**, has **lost her appetite for food and her interest in sex**, and has been **oversleeping** every day. She recently told her husband that she was **unsure whether she wanted to go on living**. She has no history of alcohol or other substance abuse.

PE PE normal; **suicidal thoughts without plan** on mental status exam.

Labs Thyroid function tests normal.

Treatment Hospitalization and supervised antidepressant therapy.

Discussion Major depressive episodes are two to three times more common in women than in men. In suicidal patients, consider an antidepressant that is safe in the event of overdose, such as selective serotonin reuptake inhibitors (SSRIs).

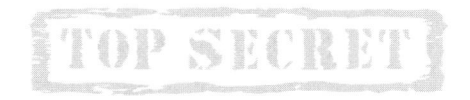

CASE 56

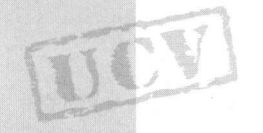

ID/CC — A 38-year-old man reveals a three-year history of **depressed mood** during a routine physical exam; he states that he is **always tired and "feeling blue."**

HPI — The patient reports that he is doing fine at work but does not hope for advancement because "I'm just not good enough." He also states, **"I don't remember ever really being happy."** The patient reports **difficulty making decisions**. Upon questioning, he denies any suicidal ideation or substance abuse.

Labs — Normal T_3, T_4, and TSH (rule out hypothyroidism).

Treatment — Some patients respond to antidepressants. Treatment should focus on insight-oriented psychotherapy and behavioral therapy.

Discussion — Patients with dysthymic disorder exhibit **chronic (2+ years) depressed mood without clear onset**. The mood is persistent (only brief periods of normal mood) and often associated with **low self-esteem, hopelessness, pessimism, and low energy**.

CASE 57

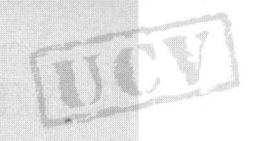

ID/CC A 30-year-old male is brought to the physician complaining that he wants to kill his fiancee's murderer and the emergency room doctors who couldn't save her.

HPI His fiancee was assaulted and died 2 days ago. During the interview, he repeatedly changes topics and talks about his fiancee's death. He frequently **alternates between apathy and anger** and **complains of vague GI discomfort** and **shortness of breath**. He also complains of **poor sleep**. He has no history of prolonged hysteria or inappropriate euphoria.

PE Patient is **restless and preoccupied** and **occasionally cries during examination; paresthesias** found that cannot be explained anatomically (SOMATIZATION DISORDER).

Treatment Medication to attenuate the normal grief process is not recommended. Small doses of **benzodiazepines for sleep** may be helpful in the short run. Patient should be allowed to grieve at his own pace. If patient is willing, he should be referred to a support group.

Discussion One-fourth of patients may experience symptoms of major depression during the first year of grief. One-tenth will have delusions or hallucinations. Some will develop somatization disorders, and others may abuse drugs or alcohol. It is differentiated from pathologic grief in that it does not cause functional or social impairment after 1 year.

MOOD DISORDERS

CASE 58

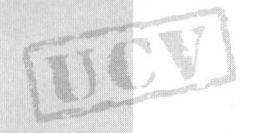

ID/CC A 55-year-old male artist complains of suffering "terrible pangs of grief" since his wife died in an auto collision 5 months ago; he claims that he is **unable to think of anything else.**

HPI The patient adds that he **has avoided most social contact** and that his art has suffered tremendously. He feels **debilitated** and wonders if he will ever emerge from his sadness.

Treatment **Grief must be differentiated from major depression**, which has similar yet more severe and prolonged symptomatology. It is important that the physician explain the normal progression of mourning, provide reassurance, and validate the patient's pain.

Discussion Pathologic grief is characterized by **intense or prolonged grief that causes functional or social impairment**, often for months. It is usually self-limited but can lead to or exacerbate chronic conditions such as depression, substance abuse, hypochondriasis, and organic disease. Distorted grief results when one aspect of grief, such as guilt, overshadows all others. Absent or delayed grief results from repression or denial of grief, which can subsequently lead to more prolonged or distorted grief.

CASE 59

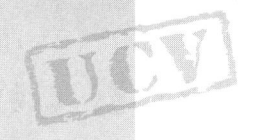

ID/CC A 26-year-old **female** presents with a sense of **bloating, swelling** of the limbs, headaches, **irritability, depression, and tension 4 days before her menses** are expected to begin.

HPI She has **similar episodes almost every month**, each **beginning 4 to 5 days prior to her menses and ending shortly after her menstrual flow begins**.

Treatment Making patients aware of the **cyclical nature** of premenstrual dysphoric disorder (PMDD) is a key part of treatment. Birth control pills (ORAL CONTRACEPTIVES) sometimes reduce the intensity of PMDD symptoms. Selective serotonin reuptake inhibitors (SSRIs) may be helpful, either continuously or in the luteal phase. Supportive psychotherapy may be beneficial.

Discussion Studies indicate that 80% of women of reproductive age experience alterations of mood and/or physical discomfort before menses (premenstrual syndrome); however, only a relatively small number (3–5%) suffer affective symptoms severe enough to result in a psychiatric diagnosis of PMDD. Diagnosis requires that symptoms occur during the **luteal phase** and a symptom-free interval begins after onset of menstruation.

MOOD DISORDERS

CASE 60

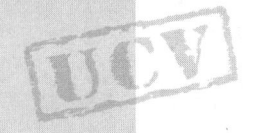

ID/CC A 32-year-old male architect is in police custody for allegedly **exposing himself** and masturbating in front of a group of people in a subway station; he admits that he often feels an **overwhelming urge to expose himself** to people he does not know, adding that he becomes **aroused by the shock in their faces**.

HPI The patient is **ashamed of his actions** but claims that he **cannot resist his impulses**. He has been **arrested** on three previous occasions over the past 10 years, each time involving self-exposure to groups of women. The patient admits that he exposes himself often, especially when he is under emotional stress.

Treatment Counseling or group therapy may help. When possible, referral to a specialist is warranted. If patient tends to expose himself to children, physician must assess the possibility that he will become more active in his sexual involvement with them.

Discussion The diagnosis of exhibitionism rests on at least a **6-month history** of **recurrent sexual fantasies or acts** that involve the **exposure of one's genitals to strangers** and cause the **patient significant distress or impairment**. It tends to be a **chronic disorder that begins during adolescence** and may decrease in severity after age 40.

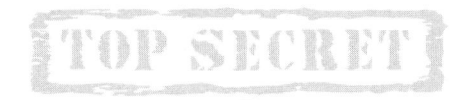

CASE 61

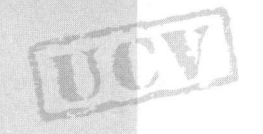

ID/CC A 22-year-old male student claims that he **uses objects of women's clothing**, especially stockings and socks, to **become sexually aroused**; he frequently masturbates while rubbing such objects, which he has stolen from various women.

HPI The patient **fears that he is "abnormal"** and that he will not be able to have a "regular" sex life because women will not understand his desires. He adds that he has **never had a sexual relationship or encounter**, although he is somewhat attracted to women. His medical history is unremarkable.

Treatment If patient is distressed about the condition, aversive conditioning, cognitive therapy, and psychotherapy may be of benefit.

Discussion The diagnosis of fetishism, a paraphilia, depends on at least a **6-month history** of recurrent sexual fantasies or acts that involve **inanimate objects** and that cause the patient significant distress or impairment. It tends to be a chronic disorder that **often begins during adolescence. Do not confuse with transvestic fetishism, which involves cross-dressing.**

PARAPHILIA

CASE 62

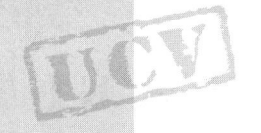

ID/CC — A 31-year-old man reveals at the end of his annual physical that he has had **recurrent urges to rub against and fondle** the buttocks of women during his daily travels on the subway.

HPI — He has occasionally followed through on these desires but **feels guilty and embarrassed** about both his actions and thoughts. His personal report and a review of his medical chart reveal no significant medical or psychiatric history. The patient is single and not sexually active, which he attributes to his shy and inhibited behavior.

Treatment — Psychotherapy employing a cognitive-behavioral framework should focus heavily on specific paraphiliac behavior. Medroxyprogesterone acetate, a testosterone antagonist, can be used as a last resort to diminish sexual drive.

Discussion — Frotteurism is diagnosed if a patient has had, over the past 6 months, **recurrent urges that involve rubbing against or touching a non-compliant person** and has **either acted on these impulses or become distressed by them**.

CASE 63

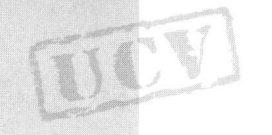

ID/CC A 49-year-old **male** teacher is placed in police custody for allegedly **undressing and fondling** one of his **10-year-old** male students; upon questioning, he reveals that he is attracted only to boys in the third-grade age group and that he has an extensive **collection of pornographic images** of **children**.

HPI The patient attempts to rationalize his behavior, saying that the boy enjoyed the experience and that it was "educational." He has long understood the social ramifications of his actions and states that he has tried many times to suppress his attractions, but to no avail. His medical history is unremarkable.

Treatment Counseling or group therapy may help. Referral to a specialist is warranted. Most states **require physicians to file reports of suspected sexual abuse of children immediately**.

Discussion Pedophilia is the most common type of paraphilia. The diagnosis can be made with a **6-month history of sexual fantasies or acts that involve sexual activity with a prepubescent child**. Varying degrees of interaction may be involved, including undressing and observing the child; exposing oneself to the child; fondling; oral-genital contact; and anal or vaginal penetration with an object, finger, or penis. The physician must gauge the likelihood that a patient will act on his fantasies.

PARAPHILIA

CASE 64

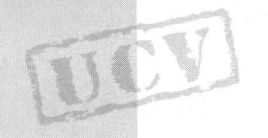

ID/CC A 32-year-old female is brought to the emergency department following a "fainting" episode; she claims that she developed dizziness and shortness of breath during sexual intercourse.

HPI Upon further questioning, she admits that her male partner, with her consent, routinely fastens a belt around her neck during intercourse, adding that she also submits routinely to being **bound, choked, and whipped** by her partner during sexual activity. She had "fantasies of being beaten and choked during sex" during adolescence but began to act on those fantasies only 2 years ago.

PE Patient alert and oriented and does not appear hypoxic; bruising around entire circumference of neck along with several horizontal scars on lower back.

Treatment If the patient is distressed about the condition, counseling or group therapy may help. Address the possible consequences of particular activities and assess the likelihood that the patient is being abused. When possible, refer to a specialist.

Discussion Sexual masochism is an example of a **paraphilia** that involves the **act of being made to suffer**. Such fantasies or acts cause the patient **significant distress, impairment, or injury**. Hypoxyphilia, in which one is oxygen-deprived by means of suffocation, strangling, or nitrate use, is a particularly dangerous form. Other forms include infantilism, physical bondage, sensory bondage (e.g., blindfolding), beating, cutting, electrical shocking, and humiliation. It tends to be a **chronic**, recurrent disorder that often begins during **early adulthood**.

CASE 65

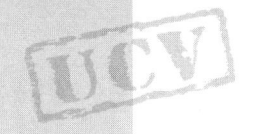

ID/CC A 30-year-old male is concerned about recurrent masturbatory **fantasies** in which he imagines himself **torturing and deriding various women**; he claims that he has never had such an encounter but that his fantasies are becoming more frequent and **violent** in nature.

HPI The patient says that he has had such fantasies for as long as he can remember but adds that they have recently become more vivid and violent, causing him to fear that he is "sick" and that he may eventually hurt someone. He imagines himself exercising complete control over a victim by binding her and whipping her into submission. The patient has had "several" female sexual partners in the past and considers himself monogamous.

Treatment Counseling, group therapy, and aversive conditioning may help. The physician should assess the risk that such patients pose to others and take appropriate action. Referral to a specialist is warranted.

Discussion Sexual sadism is an example of a **paraphilia** that involves **fantasies or acts** in which the **infliction of physical or emotional suffering is sexually arousing** to the patient. Such fantasies or acts cause the patient **significant distress or impairment**. Such acts may include humiliation, domination, physical bondage, sensory deprivation, beating, cutting, burning, electrical shocks, mutilation, rape, and killing. They may involve consenting or nonconsenting individuals. This tends to be a **chronic disorder that may begin in early childhood** and may become increasingly severe.

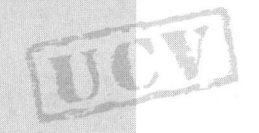

CASE 66

ID/CC A 22-year-old **male** is brought to a physician for evaluation after **committing multiple crimes** and **attempting suicide**.

HPI As a child he was hyperactive, did poorly in school, got into fights, abused animals, and was neglected by his drug-abusing parents. After dropping out of high school, he failed to hold down any job for an extended period of time and committed numerous crimes to support his drinking habit. He states that his suicide attempt was an impulsive act but adds that he **does not care what happens to him or anyone else**. He **feels no remorse** for the pain he has inflicted on others.

PE Numerous scars from fights and accidents.

Treatment Inpatient psychotherapy with confrontation and group therapy are treatment of choice.

Discussion Antisocial personality disorder is characterized by an **inability to conform to social norms** as well as by **repetitive criminal behavior**. Males are three times more likely to be affected than females.

CASE 67

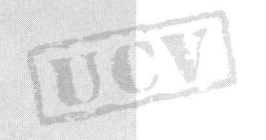

ID/CC A 23-year-old male complains of having too few friends and an **unreasonable fear of new experiences**.

HPI He reports that his **shyness** has frequently prevented him from participating in social activities. At times, his fear of criticism has affected his performance in school.

Treatment Group therapy can help.

Discussion People with avoidant personality disorder often have social phobia as well. They are **sensitive to rejection, socially withdrawn**, and **shy**. Avoidant personality disorder can be differentiated from schizoid personality disorder in that schizoid individuals are happy being alone, whereas avoidant individuals are **distressed at the prospect of being alone**.

CASE 68

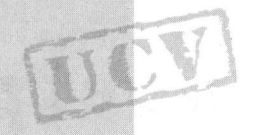

ID/CC During a routine physical exam, a young female patient tells her physician that she has **fallen in love with him**; when he recommends that she see another physician, she **threatens to commit suicide**.

HPI She denies any depression or suicidal ideation in the past. However, she does report a history of multiple, short, intense relationships. The patient ended these relationships because of fear of abandonment. She also has a history of drug abuse.

Treatment Psychiatric consultation and behavioral psychotherapy can be effective over time.

Discussion Characteristics of such a personality disorder include **unstable mood and behavior, suicide attempts, boredom, splitting, feelings of emptiness and loneliness**, and **impulsiveness**. This personality disorder is three times more common in females than in males.

CASE 69

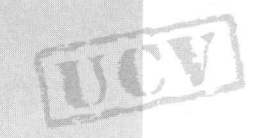

PERSONALITY DISORDERS

ID/CC A 49-year-old female homemaker complains of disillusionment with her marriage and general sadness; she states that she **feels insecure when left on her own** and has great **difficulty asserting herself**.

HPI She adds that she considers herself a "**follower**" who has always **left all decision making to her husband**. She describes her husband as an intense and domineering man who makes many demands. She has few friends other than the acquaintances she has met through her husband.

Treatment Counseling and group therapy may help. Training in assertiveness and in developing social skills may also be of value.

Discussion Dependent personality disorder denotes a **chronic, excessive dependence on others**. Such patients frequently **defer decision making** to others, **tolerate mistreatment, place others' needs before their own**, and have **difficulty being assertive**. Patients may also demonstrate **low self-esteem, insecurity, and a longing to be in a relationship**.

CASE 70

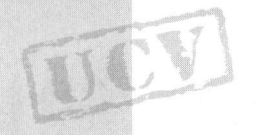

ID/CC A 27-year-old, **charming, scantily clad woman** complains of suicidal feelings and **vague musculoskeletal pain**; she asks to see "the best doctor in the hospital."

HPI She explains how she is **annoyed by a coworker who has become the center of attention at the office**. The patient **behaves seductively** and exhibits inappropriately **dramatic emotions** while omitting important details in her responses. She has a history of multiple suicide attempts, after which she claims to have **received sympathy from a multitude of "close friends."**

PE Small, shallow scars on wrists from past suicide attempts.

Treatment Patients with minor impairment can be treated with psychotherapy.

Discussion Histrionic personality disorder has a 2% prevalence in the overall population and has significant comorbidity with depression, substance abuse, and somatization disorder. People suffering from this personality disorder are **dramatic, extroverted, and emotional; exhibit sexually provocative behavior**; and are unable to maintain intimate relationships (although they often **overstate the closeness of their friendships**). These patients are often fundamentally insecure, and their theatrics are generally efforts to obtain love, support, and reassurance. Cluster B personality disorder.

CASE 71

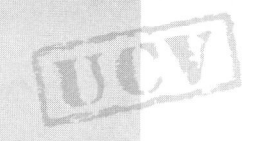

PERSONALITY DISORDERS

ID/CC A 45-year-old man is admitted to the medical unit following a heart attack; a psych consult is requested when nurses report that his **offensive behavior** is disrupting the staff and other patients.

HPI When questioned, the patient is dismissive and prefers instead to discuss his "beautiful girlfriend," new sports car, and **widespread influence**. He denies having had a heart attack and claims that it was just "minor heartburn." He loudly belittles the staff for being inattentive and claims that the consulting physician is "the only one here who can appreciate me."

Labs ECG and labs consistent with diagnosis of myocardial infarction.

Treatment Patients benefit from psychotherapy but must be **treated with sensitivity and empathy,** as confronting these difficult issues may be perceived as humiliating.

Discussion Patients with narcissistic personality disorder will often **ignore or deny illness** to protect their fragile self-esteem. These patients often have a **poor sense of self**; they compensate by **soliciting attention and praise** from others and by creating an **image of power, wealth, and attractiveness**. They often **lack empathy and exhibit a strong sense of entitlement.** They cope best with a medical setting in which they feel appreciated and admired. Cluster B personality disorder.

CASE 72

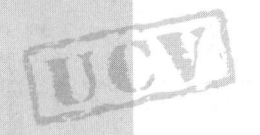

ID/CC　　A 34-year-old **male** complains of anxiety over not doing his work well enough along with an inability to enjoy recreational activities that he himself has organized.

HPI　　He describes **making lists and protocols**, and he remarks about how well he is able to organize activities. He has few friends because **work occupies most of his time**. He tends to be very thrifty and **adheres rigidly to moral and ethical values**. People often find it difficult to work with him because he is slow and **meticulous** and **demands perfection** of his coworkers.

Treatment　　Long-term psychotherapy is of benefit.

Discussion　　Obsessive-compulsive personality disorder affects males twice as often as females. Cluster C personality disorder.

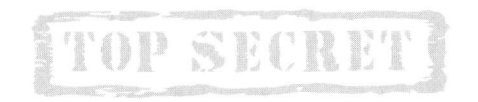

CASE 73

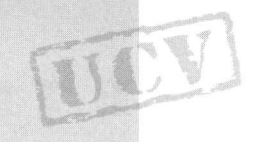

ID/CC A 55-year-old male **insists that his physician has deliberately prescribed harmful drugs for him** and states that he will file a malpractice suit against the doctor.

HPI The patient is **hostile** and angry.

PE Physical examination normal, although patient is suspicious and guarded.

Treatment Patients may benefit from supportive therapy. Medical management should include clear explanations of procedures and medications.

Discussion A patient with paranoid personality disorder is characteristically **suspicious and mistrustful, interpreting the motives of others as malevolent**. He often holds others responsible for his problems. Cluster A personality disorder.

CASE 74

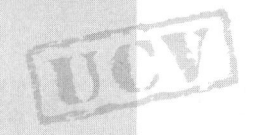

ID/CC A 48-year-old obese diabetic woman consults a physician for help in dieting, after which the doctor prepares a diet for her and discusses it with her in detail.

HPI The patient **misses her next two follow-up appointments** and does not return calls from the office staff. She eventually returns for another visit but is **30 minutes late**. She has **gained some weight** but claims that she has followed the diet regimen.

Treatment **Insight-oriented therapy** may help these patients express anger and frustration in a more direct manner. Physicians should try to involve such patients more actively in planning their medical treatment.

Discussion Characteristics of passive-aggressive personality disorder include **procrastination, stubbornness, inefficiency, and passive resistance to authority and responsibility**. This disorder is no longer recognized in DSM-IV.

CASE 75

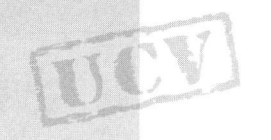

ID/CC A 40-year-old **scientist** presents for a work physical, where questioning reveals that he has **no contact with his family, does not maintain any friendships**, and lives alone.

HPI The patient **seems apathetic** with regard to his apparent dearth of social support structures. He has **never engaged in dating or other social activities**. He prefers to work alone at home and **cannot name any hobbies or activities that he finds enjoyable**.

Treatment Behavioral therapy targeting social integration may be useful.

Discussion **A lifelong pattern of voluntary social withdrawal without psychosis** is characteristic of patients suffering from schizoid personality disorder. Cluster A personality disorder.

CASE 76

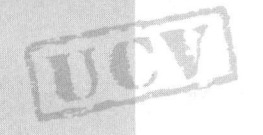

ID/CC A 38-year-old woman presents to a local clinic complaining that her left hand has disappeared.

HPI The patient is wearing **mismatched shoes** and has **colored her eyebrows with red lipstick**. When the physician examines her hands, she suddenly seems relieved and thanks him for restoring her missing hand. The patient lives alone and reports that she **avoids family and neighbors because they "can't be trusted."** She also claims that she can read others' minds.

PE Inappropriate affect; odd appearance; no hallucinations or delusions.

Treatment Low-dose neuroleptics may alleviate the social anxiety, peculiar thought patterns, and perceptual illusions of schizotypal patients. Supportive therapy can be used to encourage patients to become involved in more social activities.

Discussion Schizotypal personality disorder is characterized by a **peculiar appearance and odd thought patterns** and behavior in the **absence of psychosis**. These patients tend to become **socially isolated**. Cluster A personality disorder.

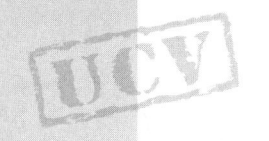

CASE 77

ID/CC A 40-year-old female high-school teacher is brought to the ER by her colleagues because they are alarmed by her odd behavior.

HPI Her coworkers noticed that she has become increasingly **anxious** of late and has begun to talk about people who are allegedly **watching her behind her back**. Her husband adds that she recently refused to get ready for bed and began pacing around the room looking in the closet and under the bed for people hiding there.

PE Patient **anxious and delusional** on mental status exam.

Labs No evidence of drug abuse on urinary screen.

Treatment Hospitalization is recommended, with an antipsychotic medication given for the acute episode.

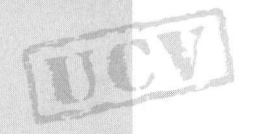

CASE 78

ID/CC A 35-year-old male tells his doctor that people at work hate him and have **conspired to eliminate him** because he complained about them to management 10 years ago.

HPI The patient's behavior and speech are normal. He denies any depression or suicidal ideation. His wife tells the physician that aside from his beliefs regarding his coworkers, he **participates normally in family activities**.

PE Neurologic exam normal; higher mental functions normal; **belief unshakable**.

Treatment Psychotherapy and antipsychotic medication can be beneficial, but delusional disorders are often refractory to treatment (vs. schizophrenia).

Discussion Delusions are **fixed and culturally inappropriate but nonbizarre beliefs** that a patient holds **despite all reasonable evidence to the contrary**. Individuals with delusional disorder have one fixed delusional system but are **otherwise relatively functional** (vs. schizophrenics).

CASE 79

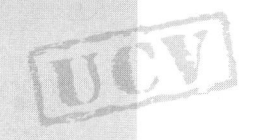

ID/CC A 73-year-old male is transferred to the ICU immediately following hip replacement surgery; on his second day in the unit, he **attempts to rise from bed** to escape the "**faces flying over his bed.**"

HPI The nurse in charge of his care reports that he has become **progressively disoriented** and has **not slept well** since his admission to the unit. He has no history of dementia.

Treatment Haloperidol, a neuroleptic, should be given as a sedative. Lorazepam can be used, although benzodiazepines may cause anterograde amnesia and may exacerbate disinhibited behavior. Treatment of underlying medical condition causing the patient's mental status change is essential.

Discussion The **disorienting environment of the hospital** often makes patients susceptible to hospital-induced psychosis or delirium.

CASE 80

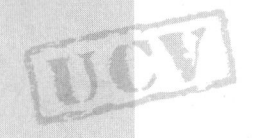

ID/CC A **20-year-old man** is brought into the ER after he was discovered trying to hang himself.

HPI The patient has become quiet and **withdrawn**, avoiding social activities and school events. His roommate reports that for the **past 6 months**, many friends have commented on his increasingly **peculiar behavior**. The roommate also reports that 2 months ago the patient began **mumbling to himself** and often pausing as if he were **listening to someone else**. Upon psychiatric evaluation, the patient **speaks in a disorganized fashion** and complains that a **voice told him to kill himself**. Further questioning reveals that the patient is still hearing the voice, which maintains a **running commentary of derisive remarks** regarding the patient's personality and actions.

Labs Drug screen negative (ruling out drug-induced psychosis).

Imaging MR, brain: normal or mild atrophy.

Treatment Neuroleptic agents can be used to control psychotic symptoms. Combining benzodiazepines with neuroleptics may be appropriate in acute situations. Hospitalization may be necessary. Long-term supportive psychotherapy along with pharmacotherapy should be utilized.

Discussion Acute schizophrenia has a 1% prevalence, with onset usually occurring in the **early 20s to 30s**. Current research suggests that schizophrenia is due to a **defect in the dopaminergic** system. Neuroleptics can cause a variety of side effects, including anticholinergic effects, postural hypertension, and tardive dyskinesia.

CASE 81

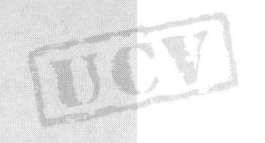

ID/CC A 22-year-old woman is brought to the psych ER by the police after she was found loitering in a large shopping mall; she is not responsive to questioning aside from an occasional parrot-like echoing of the interviewer's words.

HPI She is **unkempt**, dirty, and wearing shorts despite near-freezing temperatures. Her mother, with whom she lives, reports that within the past 2 years the patient has become increasingly "sullen" and has periods during which she "**refuses to speak or even budge.**" The mother has also noticed that the patient often speaks in a loose, tangential fashion. The mother complains that she is too busy to pay attention to her daughter's problems but nonetheless claims that her daughter is just "going through a phase." The patient recently withdrew from her classes at the local college.

PE **Posture fairly rigid** throughout examination; patient's limbs maintain various positions induced by physician during exam (WAXY FLEXIBILITY OR CATALEPSY).

Labs Drug/EtOH screen negative.

Treatment Treat schizophrenia; patients should also be carefully monitored to prevent self-injury or malnutrition.

Discussion Patients with catatonic schizophrenia may exhibit peculiar voluntary movements, grimacing, senseless repetition of words spoken by another (ECHOLALIA), and repetitive imitation of another person's movements (ECHOPRAXIA). General medical disorders, substance abuse, and major depression must be ruled out.

CASE 82

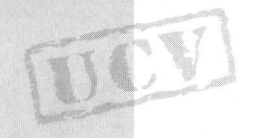

ID/CC: A thin, **poorly groomed 25-year-old man** is brought to the ER by a concerned neighbor who claims that the patient stopped going to work 3 weeks ago and often speaks in a **nonsensical, discontinuous fashion**; she strongly suspects alcohol abuse but can find no evidence of it in his household.

HPI: The neighbor also states that within the past year the patient has exhibited **increasingly "bizarre" behavior**, such as failing to wash himself, maintain his appearance, or eat properly. Once friendly and talkative, the patient now avoids other people and spends hours cutting shapes out of the newspaper. The patient attempts to answer the physician's questions but is quickly sidetracked, frequently lapsing into **silence or incoherence**. His **speech is difficult to follow** and is often punctuated by laughing or giggling that is seemingly unrelated to the subject at hand.

Labs: Drug/EtOH screen negative.

Treatment: As with other types of schizophrenia, this patient may respond to neuroleptic medications combined with long-term supportive psychotherapy.

Discussion: Patients with the disorganized subtype of schizophrenia exhibit **disorganized speech, disorganized behavior, and flat/inappropriate affect**. Their lack of goal orientation may affect their ability to perform activities of daily living.

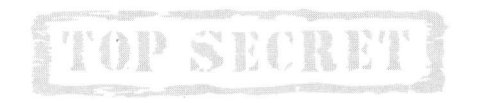

CASE 83

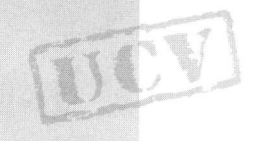

ID/CC A 17-year-old man is brought by his parents to the psych ER because they have been increasingly alarmed by his **suspicious** and unpredictable demeanor over the past 6 months.

HPI The patient reveals to the interviewing psychiatrist that he believes his parents are **trying to kill him**. He also explains that he read an article in the local paper which he has interpreted to mean that somebody is trying **to warn him of the danger**. His teachers have observed that the patient has become much more **withdrawn** and socializes less frequently with his classmates.

Labs Drug/EtOH screen negative.

Treatment As with other types of schizophrenia, this patient may respond to neuroleptic medications combined with long-term supportive psychotherapy.

Discussion Despite treatment with neuroleptics and supportive psychotherapy, patients with paranoid schizophrenia may never regain their former level of functioning.

CASE 84

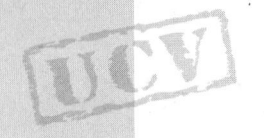

ID/CC A 35-year-old woman with an extensive psychiatric history comes to her internist's office wearing three large skirts layered over a pair of pants despite the mild summer weather; she denies having hallucinations or hearing voices but explains that her deceased mother warned her to dress warmly.

HPI The patient **speaks in a loose, tangential fashion and occasionally lapses into incoherent speech.** She has been hospitalized six times for inability to care for herself and acute psychosis. During these episodes, she experienced vivid visual hallucinations involving various deceased family members and expressed the belief that those family members wanted to kill her. **Her last hospitalization was 3 years ago.**

Labs Drug/EtOH screen negative.

Treatment Neuroleptics, antidepressants, and supportive psychotherapy.

Discussion The diagnosis of residual-type schizophrenia can be made if **negative symptoms are still present or if patients present with two positive symptoms (delusions, hallucinations, disorganized speech, or grossly disorganized/catatonic behavior) in attenuated form.**

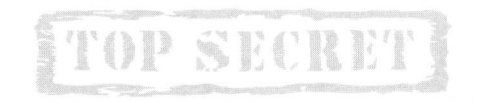

CASE 85

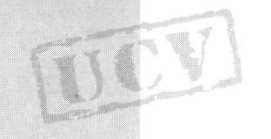

ID/CC A 29-year-old woman presents for a follow-up visit following a 3-week **remission from a 4-month period of psychotic episodes.**

HPI During that 4-month period, the patient **heard voices** conversing with one another and suspected that her mind **was being controlled by a voice on the radio.** These auditory hallucinations were much more intrusive in the morning. The patient attempted to drown out the voices by listening to a Walkman and managed to maintain marginal performance at her nighttime cleaning job. At the time of this visit, the patient denies hearing any voices and no longer holds the delusion of mind control, reporting that her performance at work has improved significantly.

Labs Lab studies normal.

Treatment During the symptomatic period, the patient may have responded to neuroleptic medications.

Discussion The diagnosis of schizophreniform disorder is based on **schizophrenia-like symptoms for more than 1 month but less than 6 months.** If the patient is symptomatic but has been so for less than 6 months, the diagnosis should be "schizophreniform—provisional." One-third of these patients recover within 6 months; the remainder progress to a diagnosis of schizophrenia.

CASE 86

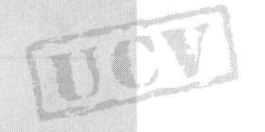

ID/CC — A 52-year-old female accountant complains that she has had **difficulty falling and staying asleep** for 2 months; she states that the sleep she does manage to get is **not restful** and that she is easily awakened by noises.

HPI — The patient adds that she is **fatigued during the day** and as a result is performing poorly at her job. She says that she has always been a "light" sleeper. She denies feeling depressed, although she admits that she gets irritable when tired. She takes no medications and drinks two cups of coffee each day, always before noon.

PE — The patient appears fatigued but is otherwise in good health.

Treatment — **Rule out other potentially precipitating disorders, especially depression. Institute sleep hygiene measures**, e.g., sleep only as much as is necessary; establish regular hours for sleep; exercise; avoid caffeine, alcohol, tobacco, and other stimulants; leave the bed when not tired. Hypnotic agents (e.g., benzodiazepines, zolpidem) may aid in short-term management.

Discussion — Complaints of insomnia are most prevalent among women and the elderly. Younger patients tend to report more difficulty in initiating sleep, while the elderly tend to have more difficulty maintaining sleep. A diagnosis of primary insomnia depends on excluding other causes. Differential diagnosis includes circadian rhythm disorder, primary hypersomnia, narcolepsy, sleep apnea, parasomnias, and sleep disorders secondary to other medical and psychiatric disorders.

CASE 87

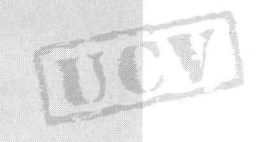

ID/CC A **12-year-old girl** is brought to her pediatrician by her parents, who report that she has been repeatedly **walking "like a zombie" in her sleep**. Twice she has walked into the closet and urinated there in her sleep.

HPI It is **difficult to awaken** the patient during these episodes, and she is **only briefly confused minutes upon awakening and does not recall the episode**. Her parents are very concerned about her inappropriate behavior and fear for her safety. Her mother adds that the patient has **begun to avoid her classmates' slumber parties** and is **reluctant to stay with relatives overnight**. They fear that she is becoming **socially isolated as a result**. The patient has no history of seizures or similar episodes during the day.

PE Physical exam normal; mental status exam unremarkable; some anxiety noted.

Treatment Parents should be reassured that sleepwalking usually disappears spontaneously during early adolescence. Sharp objects and obstacles should be removed from the floor. A course of short-acting benzodiazepines or tricyclic antidepressants may be useful in conjunction with psychotherapy.

Discussion Somnambulism occurs in delta sleep, usually during the first third of the night. Sleepwalking disorder in adults warrants psychiatric evaluation. Post-traumatic stress disorder, acute stress disorder, and somatoform disorder should be part of the differential.

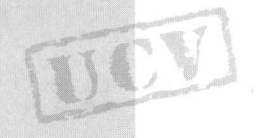

CASE 88

ID/CC A **17-year-old woman** in her first year of college presents to the student health services with complaints of fever and sore throat.

HPI Careful questioning reveals that the patient is not physically ill but rather made up the story out of reluctance to admit her desire to see if "someone can do something about my lips." She states that her **lips "are too fat"** and that their appearance **impedes her ability to socialize normally with her peers.** Her embarrassment has progressed to such a degree that she no longer attends her classes.

PE Physical exam reveals a healthy and attractive young woman.

Treatment Psychiatric intervention using group or individual therapy and focusing on psychosocial functions and body image has proven effective. SSRIs may be helpful in controlling obsessional thinking.

Discussion Body dysmorphic disorder is **characterized by a preoccupation with an imagined defect in appearance that causes clinically significant distress or impairment in social, occupational, or other important areas of functioning** and excludes any other mental disorder. Some researchers regard this syndrome as a prodrome of schizophrenia.

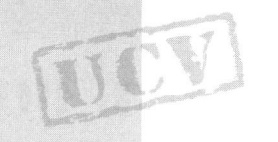

CASE 89

ID/CC A 26-year-old female is brought to her family physician with complaints of an **inability to speak or to move** the right side of body for the past hour.

HPI She **received news of the death** of her 3-year-old child **immediately before the onset of her symptoms**. Her previous history, as elicited from her spouse, suggests an **underlying dependent personality disorder**. She comes from a rural background and is not well educated.

PE **Fundus, pupils, deep tendon reflexes normal**; mutism noted; "la belle indifférence" to symptoms.

Treatment Psychotherapy used to detect underlying conflict and repressed thoughts; emotional release sought through hypnosis.

Discussion Conversion disorder is a **type of somatoform disorder**.

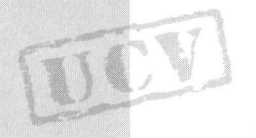

CASE 90

ID/CC — A 23-year-old medical student complains of abdominal pain that has lasted for over 6 months.

HPI — The patient **believes that his abdominal pain is indicative of a serious illness**. Although previous medical examinations by several other physicians found **no serious pathology**, he continues to believe that he has a severe medical problem. **His preoccupation with the "disease"** has begun to interfere with his social and occupational activities.

PE — Poorly localized abdominal tenderness.

Labs — Routine laboratory studies normal.

Treatment — Telling the patient that no pathology exists is often futile; best results are achieved by helping patient cope with perceived illness.

Discussion — Hypochondriasis must be differentiated from somatization disorders, anxiety disorders, and depressive disorders. If any of these disorders is present, treatment of the underlying condition will often lead to the resolution of hypochondriasis.

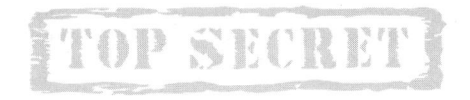

CASE 91

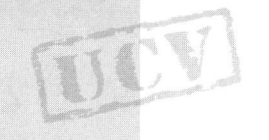

ID/CC A 30-year-old **male** complains of **persistent inability to maintain an erection during intercourse.**

HPI He states that his disorder is causing difficulty in his marriage. He has no history of psychiatric disorder and **denies any drug or medication use.** He has no acute or chronic illness and no history of genitourinary surgery.

PE VS: BP normal.

Labs Lytes: normal. Testosterone, TSH, LH, FSH, and prolactin normal; **nocturnal penile tumescence reveals erection** during REM sleep.

Treatment **Individual and couples therapy is treatment of choice.** If a medication can be implicated, it should be changed. Once organic pathology has been excluded, pharmacotherapy with sildenafil may help.

Discussion Almost **90%** of male erectile dysfunction is believed to be of **psychogenic origin**. Medication- and acute illness-induced erectile dysfunction can also occur. Substances known to cause erectile dysfunction include some tricyclic antidepressants, MAO inhibitors, anticholinergics, ethanol, and amphetamines. Disorders of the hypothalamic-pituitary axis, thyroid, and kidneys must be ruled out.

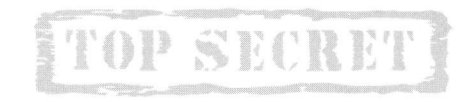

SOMATOFORM DISORDERS

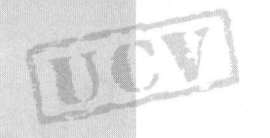

CASE 92

ID/CC — A 29-year-old woman presents to her family physician following a **positive home-pregnancy test**.

HPI — She reports an 8-week history of amenorrhea accompanied by breast tenderness, malaise, lassitude, and nausea. A repeat **pregnancy test in the doctor's office is positive for hCG**. The patient is elated because she has been trying to become pregnant for 1 year.

PE — Weight gain of 4 pounds in 6 weeks; uterus soft and enlarged; cervix soft and cyanotic.

Imaging — US, uterus: at week 13 shows **empty uterine cavity without any evidence of fetal parts or gestational sac**; no evidence of ectopic pregnancy.

Discussion — False pregnancy (PSEUDOCYESIS) can manifest with many of the physical signs and symptoms of pregnancy. It may occur in women who have a strong desire to be pregnant or in women with a strong fear of pregnancy.

CASE 93

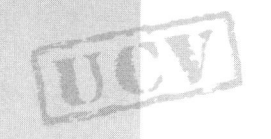

ID/CC A 36-year-old **woman** presents to the ER with a 2-day history of progressive right lower quadrant pain.

HPI A review of systems reveals **numerous symptoms**. Further questioning reveals that she has been sickly since **early adolescence** with numerous chronic symptoms, including **nausea, bloating, polyarticular joint pain, dyspareunia, dysmenorrhea, and difficulty swallowing**. She is **frustrated with her many ailments** and by **her failure to find a medical explanation for them** despite visits to numerous physicians. The patient also reveals that she has been feeling "very stressed out" due to an impending divorce and her mother's recent death.

PE Physical exam reveals no abnormalities.

Labs No leukocytosis.

Treatment Treatment should include employment of therapeutic alliance, scheduling of regular appointments, and crisis intervention utilizing psychiatric consult services. Prognostic outlook is fair. These individuals are often highly resistant to psychiatric referral.

Discussion Differential diagnosis includes physical disease and depression. The onset of somatization disorder occurs before age 30. Almost 1% of all women are affected. There is a 20% concordance rate for first-degree female relatives. Symptoms **are not intentionally feigned** or produced (vs. factitious disorder).

SOMATOFORM DISORDERS

CASE 94

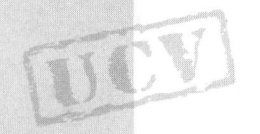

ID/CC	A 20-year-old female complains of **severe pain** that **prevents her from attaining the social and occupational goals** she has set for herself.
HPI	The patient receives temporary relief with physical therapy, but the pain inevitably returns some time later. **Stress tends to exacerbate the pain.**
PE	The pain does not follow any anatomic distribution.
Labs	Physical examination normal.
Treatment	Counseling with goal of improving coping strategies is primary treatment; judicious use of antidepressants and anxiolytics may also help.
Discussion	Confronting patients with somatoform disorder may worsen symptoms.

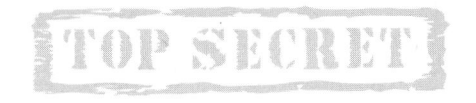

CASE 95

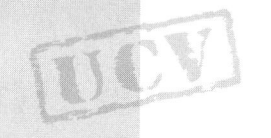

ID/CC A 27-year-old woman presenting for her annual gynecologic exam reveals that she has been unable to participate in sexual intercourse because of **severe vaginal contractions** elicited by attempts at penile penetration of the vagina.

HPI Further questioning reveals that the patient has experienced these symptoms many times in the past with various sexual partners. She has been dating her current partner for 4 months and has become progressively anxious with respect to their heightened sexual activity; **she wishes to have intercourse** with him yet fears a repetition of past failures. She also reports difficulty in inserting tampons.

PE Genital examination incomplete because of **inability to insert speculum**.

Treatment Successful treatment is based in behavioral methods that desensitize patient to experience of penetration. Systematic insertion of dilators of graduated sizes, either at the physician's office or in the privacy of the patient's home, may be helpful.

Discussion The contractions are **involuntary reflex spasms of the muscles of the vagina**. Vaginismus is **sometimes secondary to genital/sexual trauma**.

CASE 96

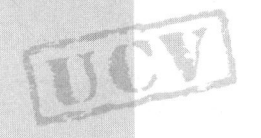

ID/CC: A successful 50-year-old business executive becomes **agitated** upon his admission to an orthopedic ward with a fractured femur; **he complains that people are making derogatory comments about him** and are accusing him of impotence (PARANOID DELUSIONS).

HPI: On persistent questioning, he admits to "moderate" alcohol intake. There is no personal, past, or family history suggestive of any major psychiatric illness.

PE: Psychomotor **agitation**; **anxious** and slightly tremulous but well oriented; remainder of neurologic, funduscopic, and systemic exam normal.

Treatment: **Haloperidol** is effective in relieving hallucinosis.

Discussion: **Auditory hallucinations** and/or **paranoid delusions** can occur with **alcohol withdrawal**, as can **anxiety** and **sadness**. Assessment of alcohol intake is an important part of the differential in any patient presenting with these symptoms.

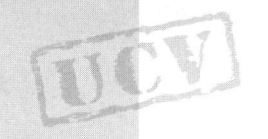

CASE 97

ID/CC A 20-year-old male is brought to the emergency room in a severely **agitated** state.

HPI According to a friend, the patient **took "angel dust"** about an hour before his arrival in the ER.

PE Patient severely agitated, **belligerent**, emotionally **labile**, and **frightened**; **speech slurred** (DYSARTHRIA); vertical and **horizontal nystagmus** noted. Diminished response to painful stimuli.

Labs UA: **phencyclidine (PCP) metabolites**.

Treatment **Diazepam and minimizing sensory stimulation** are useful in controlling agitated state.

Discussion PCP can induce a psychosis similar to schizophrenia. It is a noncompetitive antagonist at the glutamate N-methyl-D-aspartate (NMDA) receptor.

ANSWER KEY

1. AIDS Dementia
2. Amnesia—Postencephalitis
3. Delirium—Inhalant Abuse
4. Delirium—Medical Cause
5. Dementia—Alzheimer's
6. Dementia—Vascular
7. Narcolepsy
8. Seizure, Absence
9. Seizure, Grand Mal
10. Seizure, Jacksonian Type
11. Seizure, Temporal Lobe
12. Status Epilepticus
13. Acting Out
14. Denial
15. Devaluation
16. Displacement
17. Fixation
18. Identification
19. Isolation of Affect
20. Rationalization
21. Reaction Formation
22. Regression
23. Repression
24. Splitting
25. Sublimation
26. Adjustment Disorder
27. Generalized Anxiety Disorder
28. Obsessive-Compulsive Disorder
29. Panic Disorder
30. Post-Traumatic Stress Disorder
31. Social Phobia
32. Attention-Deficit Hyperactivity Disorder
33. Autism
34. Child Abuse—Shaken Baby Syndrome
35. Conduct Disorder
36. Enuresis
37. Post-Traumatic Stress Disorder
38. Separation Anxiety
39. Sleep Terrors
40. Tic Disorders—Tourette's
41. Dissociative Amnesia
42. Dissociative Disorder (Depersonalization)
43. Dissociative Fugue
44. Dissociative Identity Disorder
45. Anorexia Nervosa
46. Bulimia Nervosa
47. Malingering
48. Munchausen's Syndrome
49. Gender Identity Disorder
50. Bipolar I Disorder, Manic Type
51. Bipolar II Disorder
52. Cyclothymic Disorder
53. Depression—Elderly
54. Depression—Suicidal
55. Depressive Episode—Major
56. Dysthymic Disorder
57. Grief—Normal
58. Grief—Pathologic
59. Premenstrual Dysphoric Disorder
60. Exhibitionism
61. Fetishism
62. Frotteurism
63. Pedophilia
64. Sexual Masochism
65. Sexual Sadism
66. Antisocial Personality Disorder
67. Avoidant Personality Disorder
68. Borderline Personality Disorder
69. Dependent Personality Disorder
70. Histrionic Personality Disorder
71. Narcissistic Personality Disorder
72. Obsessive-Compulsive Personality Disorder
73. Paranoid Personality Disorder
74. Passive-Aggressive Personality Disorder
75. Schizoid Personality Disorder
76. Schizotypal Personality Disorder
77. Brief Psychotic Episode
78. Delusional Disorder
79. ICU Psychosis
80. Schizophrenia—Acute
81. Schizophrenia—Catatonic
82. Schizophrenia—Disorganized
83. Schizophrenia—Paranoid
84. Schizophrenia—Residual
85. Schizophreniform Disorder
86. Primary Insomnia
87. Sleepwalking Disorder

- **88.** Body Dysmorphic Disorder
- **89.** Conversion Disorder
- **90.** Hypochondriasis
- **91.** Male Erectile Disorder—Psychogenic
- **92.** Pseudocyesis
- **93.** Somatization Disorder
- **94.** Somatoform Pain Disorder
- **95.** Vaginismus
- **96.** Alcoholic Hallucinosis
- **97.** PCP Intoxication

QUESTIONS

1. A test for a disease X is known to have a sensitivity of 0.95, specificity of 0.65, positive predictive value of 0.73, and a negative predictive value of 0.93. What is the false negative rate?

    A: 0.05
    B: 0.08
    C: 0.27
    D: 0.35
    E: Undeterminable from the information given.

2. You see a patient in a locked in-patient psychiatric ward at 7 AM. He wears a long formal overcoat, a top hat, walks with a straight black cane, and wears bright pink bunny slippers and a matched bright pink shirt. Before even speaking to this gentleman, you think it most likely he has which of the following disorders:

    A: Antisocial
    B: Borderline
    C: Paranoid
    D: Schizoid
    E: Schizotypal

3. While on your psychiatric rotation you are assigned a bipolar patient to follow. You review all of your patient's medications and medical records. You are concerned because you do not believe adequate monitoring labs have been obtained on this patient. In addition to obtaining levels for the drug of choice for long-term prophylaxis for bipolar disorder, which laboratory values would you most like to obtain with regard to this medication?

    A: Cardiac enzymes due to the drug's effect on the myocardium.
    B: Complete blood count because this drug causes agranulocytosis.
    C: Thyroid stimulating hormone and blood urea nitrogen (BUN)
    D: Thyroid stimulating hormone and creatinine
    E: Thyroid stimulating hormone and complete blood count

4. A nurse calls you to the pediatric floor to evaluate a 14-month-old child for vomiting. The child was admitted four days ago with complaints of persistent vomiting at home. The nurse states the child slept peacefully through the night and began vomiting around 11 AM. You review the medical record and note a suspicious pattern to the vomiting since the child's admission. The vomiting usually starts within one hour of the start of visiting hours and seems to occur only when the child's mother is visiting. It does not occur when the father visits or other family members are visiting. You suspect:

    A: Munchausen's syndrome and the mother is the culprit.
    B: Munchausen's syndrome by proxy and the mother is the culprit.
    C: This child has been physically abused by the mother and the vomiting is a stress reaction by the child to the mother's presence.

101

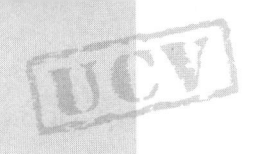

D: The child's mother is carrying an infectious agent that keeps reinfecting the child every time she visits.

E: The child is vomiting in front of the mother because he knows he will get extra attention from this behavior.

5. A 32-year-old man who is a frequent visitor to the emergency room when it is cold outside. He is known panhandler who drinks himself to sleep at night. He says that drinking is his way of calming the voices in his head. He has never been known to be violent. He does not seem to be malnourished. He refuses anti-psychotic medication. Should he be admitted involuntarily?

   A: Yes, he needs to be detoxed from the alcohol.
   B: Yes, he needs some antipsychotic medication.
   C: Yes, all homeless people who are mentally ill should be hospitalized.
   D: No, but he can be offered a non-psychiatric hospital stay.
   E: No, but he can be offered a psychiatric/detox hospital stay.

6. A 7-year-old child with cerebral palsy is more affected on the left side. His right arm is placed in a plaster cast for one month to allow his left arm to become more functional. This is thought to work through brain plasticity. The casting of his more functional arm is what kind of prevention?

   A: Primary
   B: Secondary
   C: Tertiary
   D: Quaternary
   E: This is not a kind of prevention.

7. A 21-year-old male college student is brought to the doctor by his parents. They report that the patient is "flunking out" of college. His friends called them because they were concerned. For the past 8 months the patient has not been going to class, and rarely leaves his room. Prior to that, the patient made above average grades and though introverted, was friendly, polite, and got along well with others. On the occasions when his friends have persuaded him to go somewhere, his behavior was odd, including announcing that he was the king and that everyone else was beneath him. His parents also report that he lost his job at a fast food restaurant 5 months ago for unpredictable behavior, failure to show up for all shifts, and disturbing the customers. You note the patient to appear disheveled and muttering under his breath. Which of the following is this patient's most likely diagnosis.

   A: Brief psychotic disorder
   B: Schizoaffective disorder
   C: Schizoid personality disorder
   D: Schizophrenia
   E: Schizophreniform disorder

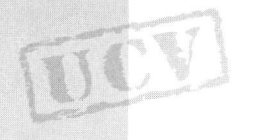

8. A 70-year-old female comes to your office complaining of the gradual development of mild forgetfulness. She describes this forgetfulness as an inability to remember phone numbers and an inability to remember the names of people that she meets. The patient is not having any problems with her activities of daily living and she is able to live independently. You perform the geriatric depressions screening questionnaire and the patient does not show signs of depression. The patient asks you what is happening to her memory. You tell the patient the following:

   A: The patient is experiencing normal aging.
   B: The patient has signs of Alzheimer's disease.
   C: The patient has pseudodementia.
   D: The patient has multi-infarct dementia.
   E: The patient's forgetfulness is most likely transient and will resolve over time.

9. While interviewing a 25-year-old male with an apparent psychotic episode, the patient reports to you that during the news last night, the news anchorwoman on television was talking about him during her broadcast on world news. He does not understand why no one else in the room picked up on it. Which of the following does this patient most likely demonstrate?

   A: Auditory hallucination
   B: Delusion
   C: Idea of reference
   D: Illusion
   E: Visual hallucination

10. The parents of a 5-year-old child report that the child repeatedly wakes up in the middle of the night screaming. The child does not recall screaming or having a nightmare. Sleep studies show that the episodes occur during delta wave sleep. The child most likely will be diagnosed with:

    A: Nightmare disorder
    B: Nocturnal myoclonus
    C: No sleep disorder
    D: Sleep terror disorder
    E: Temporal lobe epilepsy

11. While reviewing a 25-year-old female's chart prior to her appointment, you note that she has schizophrenia with positive symptoms only. Which of the following is she most likely to exhibit?

    A: Cognitive disturbances
    B: Delusions
    C: Flattened affect
    D: Poor grooming
    E: Social withdrawal
    F: Thought blocking

103

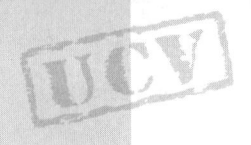

12. You have just admitted a 16-year-old female with a diagnosis of anorexia nervosa to the hospital for treatment. Which of the following characteristics is this patient most likely to exhibit?

    A: Dental caries
    B: Electrolyte disturbances
    C: From a low socioeconomic group
    D: High academic achievement
    E: Swelling of parotid and salivary glands

13. An 18-year-old female presents following an overdose of acetaminophen. She tells you that life has gotten too difficult and she just can't take it any more. Which of the following is true regarding suicide in the United States?

    A: Women successfully commit suicide four times more often than men.
    B: Approximately 75% of people who attempt suicide once will try again.
    C: The suicide rate in the U.S. is about 50 per 100,000.
    D: Suicide is the eighth leading cause of death.
    E: There are about four times more suicide attempts than actual suicides.

14. A 14-year-old girl has excessive, virtually daily anxieties about her school activities for the last year. The patient comes to see you when she has got so much anxiety that she is unable to function in school. What do you do?

    A: Prescribe Haldol.
    B: Prescribe Wellbutrin.
    C: Prescribe Lorazepam initially, then Haldol.
    D: Prescribe Lorazepam initially, then Wellbutrin.
    E: Prescribe ECT.

15. A 25-year-old woman presents to the psychiatrist with her exasperated husband. He reports that her mood swings are getting to be too much to bear. He states that last week, she did not sleep at all, staying awake at night cleaning, dancing, and watching television. He also reports that she went on a $5000 shopping spree, which exceeds what their budget allows. He states that she had a similar episode 6 months ago. Which of the following is this patient's most likely diagnosis?

    A: Major depressive disorder
    B: Bipolar I disorder
    C: Bipolar II disorder
    D: Cyclothymic disorder
    E: Dysthymic disorder

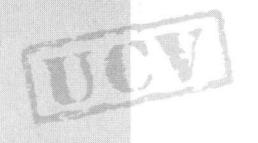

16. The attributable risk with exposure to an environmental toxin is 0.9. It is known that the disease risk in unexposed groups is 0.01. What is the relative risk?

    A: 0.81
    B: 9
    C: 90
    D: 91
    E: 900

17. A 28-year-old female presents to her primary care doctor. She states that she is in a relationship and that some of the things she does really bothers her boyfriend. These things include her constant worry over her apartment, including vacuuming the carpet at least twice per day, dusting every day, and cleaning the toilet following every use. She also washes her hands so many times a day that her skin is very dry and flaky. She sees no problem with her behavior and just wants to avoid each and every germ that she may possibly contact. Which of the following disorder does she most likely have?

    A: Adjustment disorder
    B: Generalized anxiety disorder
    C: Obsessive-compulsive disorder
    D: Panic disorder
    E: Social phobia

18. A 43-year-old woman calls you for treatment of her morbid obesity. She is afraid to leave the house and refuses to take pills thinking that evil little men from Mars make all the pills in the world. She is oriented to her surroundings and functions adequately with meals on wheels and weekly visits from her family. The only treatment you know of is an experimental shot for this condition. Can this patient participate in the study?

    A: Psychotic patients cannot participate in research experiments.
    B: Psychotic patients can participate in research experiments.
    C: Being psychotic bears no relation to participation in research protocols.
    D: Her family should be consulted for permission.
    E: The patient should be convinced to leave her house for treatment.

19. A neurologist wishes to test a child's developmental age. He takes two glasses of equal sizes, filled to the same level. The child is satisfied that the glasses are identical. Now, with the child watching, he pours the water in one of the glasses into a smaller, fatter glass. What is the first age would a developmentally average child say that there is same amount of water in both glasses?

    A: 4
    B: 5
    C: 6
    D: 7
    E: 8

105

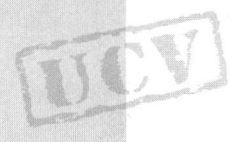

20. Which of the following is primary preventative care?
    - A: Doing PSA tests for all men at the VA hospital
    - B: Doing yearly Pap smears
    - C: Giving antihypertensive medication to someone with hypertension
    - D: Giving MMR vaccination to a child
    - E: Testing a diabetic for peripheral neuropathy

ANSWERS

1. A

    A: 0.05 [Correct]
    B: 0.08 [Incorrect] This is 1-negative predictive value. This would be the probability of having the condition given a negative test.
    C: 0.27 [Incorrect] This is 1-positive predictive value. This would be the probability of not having the condition given a positive test.
    D: 0.35 [Incorrect] The false positive ratio is 1-specificity or 0.35. This is the probability of testing positive for the disease among all the people who do not have the disease.
    E: Undeterminable from the information given. [Incorrect] The false negative rate is the ratio of people who test negative among all the people who have the disease. Thus, this is 1-sensitivity or 0.05.

2. E

    A: Antisocial. [Incorrect] Antisocial patients do not care about the norms of society and will do what they please.
    B: Borderline. [Incorrect] Borderline patients vacillate between objects and people being all good or all bad.
    C: Paranoid. [Incorrect] Paranoid patients characteristically have suspiciousness and are very distrustful of people around them.
    D: Schizoid. [Incorrect] Schizoid patients voluntarily choose to withdraw socially.
    E: Schizotypal. [Correct] Schizotypal patients have bizarre thoughts and appearance.

3. D

    A: Cardiac enzymes due to the drug's effect on the myocardium. [Incorrect] Lithium, at toxic levels can cause coma and cardiac arrest. Monitoring cardiac enzymes would not be an effective way to check for this complication.
    B: Complete blood count because this drug causes agranulocytosis. [Incorrect] Clozapine causes agranulocytosis and is not the drug of choice for bipolar disorder. Clozapine is an atypical antipsychotic.
    C: Thyroid stimulating hormone and blood urea nitrogen (BUN). [Incorrect] Lithium has been known to cause alterations in thyroid function and kidney function. Thyroid stimulating hormone would be the best way to monitor thyroid function but kidney function is best measured by creatinine. Any alteration in kidney function could lead to toxic levels of lithium which has a very narrow therapeutic index.
    D: Thyroid stimulating hormone and creatinine. [Correct] Thyroid stimulating hormone would be the best way to monitor thyroid function and kidney function is best measured by creatinine. Any alteration in kidney function could lead to toxic levels of lithium which has a very narrow therapeutic index.

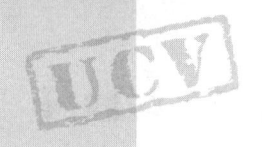

E: Thyroid stimulating hormone and complete blood count. [Incorrect]

4. B

A: Munchausen's syndrome and the mother is the culprit. [Incorrect] Munchausen's syndrome is an extreme form of a factious disorder where an individual creates or feigns an illness. They are generally pathological liars and they tend to wander. These individuals are usually younger women of middle to upper middle class status who are well educated and may work in a medically related profession.

B: Munchausen's syndrome by proxy and the mother is the culprit. [Correct] This case has all the makings of a Munchausen's syndrome by proxy. The child only seems to become ill when the mother is present. This disorder usually involves a parent or caregiver inducing an illness in a child. This is done to obtain attention for the caregiver. The caregiver has a psychological need for the child to assume the "sick role." As with Munchausen's syndrome the caregiver tends to be a female (though males have also been known to be perpetrators), in their 20s or 30s, and of middle to upper middle class status. Munchausen's syndrome by proxy is a form of child abuse and the child welfare authorities should be notified.

C: This child has been physically abused by the mother and the vomiting is a stress reaction by the child to the mother's presence. [Incorrect] It is highly unlikely that a 14-month-old child would manifest vomiting as a stress reaction to an abuser. Such a child may withdraw from the abuser or cry/whimper in their presence.

D: The child's mother is carrying an infectious agent that keeps reinfecting the child every time she visits. [Incorrect] An infectious etiology would not present in this way; starting when the mother arrives and ending with her departure.

E: The child is vomiting in front of the mother because he knows he will get extra attention from this behavior. [Incorrect] The answer implies that the child is feigning illness to obtain attention. This behavior would not manifest itself in a 14-month-old child.

5. E

A: Yes, he needs to be detoxed from the alcohol. [Incorrect] He has never been known to be violent and does not appear malnourished. A patient can only be admitted for a risk to harm himself or others. There is no evidence of this at this time.

B: Yes, he needs some antipsychotic medication. [Incorrect] A patient can only be forced to receive antipsychotic medication with a court order if he refuses.

C: Yes, all homeless people who are mentally ill should be hospitalized. [Incorrect] In many states, the loss of federal funding led to the discharge of many mentally ill who were ill equipped for the normal world and are homeless. This has led to the behavior of some patients going from hospital to hospital for a place to sleep.

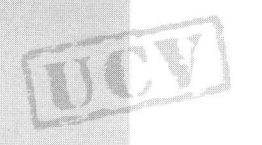

D: No, but he can be offered a non-psychiatric hospital stay. [Incorrect] There is no indication that the patient has a medical problem.

E: No, but he can be offered a psychiatric/detox hospital stay. [Correct] This can be offered to possibly help the patient improve his life.

6. C

A: Primary. [Incorrect] Primary prevention is preventing a disease or a condition from happening at all. An example would be a vaccination.

B: Secondary. [Incorrect] Secondary prevention is the early detection of a disease. It would include screening for colon cancer.

C: Tertiary. [Correct] Tertiary prevention is mitigating the effects of a disease or condition once the disease or condition is established and unable to be cured. Casting the right arm to improve the more affected left arm therefore is an example of tertiary prevention.

D: Quaternary. [Incorrect] There is no such thing as quaternary prevention.

E: This is not a kind of prevention. [Incorrect] Not a correct answer if it fits the definition of tertiary prevention.

7. D

A: Brief psychotic disorder [Incorrect] In brief psychotic disorder, the symptoms last less than 1 month and greater than 1 day. This patient has been having problems much longer than that.

B: Schizoaffective disorder [Incorrect] Patients with schizoaffective disorder have symptoms of a mood disorder in addition to psychotic symptoms.

C: Schizoid personality disorder [Incorrect] Schizoid personality disorder consists of social withdrawal without the presence of psychosis.

D: Schizophrenia [Correct] The above patient most likely has schizophrenia. His psychotic symptoms have lasted longer than 6 months and he appears to have chronic occupational and social impairment.

E: Schizophreniform disorder [Incorrect] In schizophreniform disorder, the symptoms last 1–6 months.

8. A

A: The patient is experiencing normal aging. [Correct] The patient is describing symptoms of normal aging such as mild forgetfulness and inability to learn new things quickly. The patient is not having difficulty with performing her activities of daily living. You would be

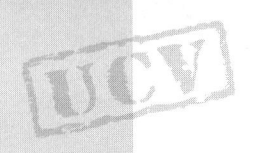

more concerned of a pathological process if the patient was having trouble with her activities of daily living.
B: The patient has signs of Alzheimer's disease. [Incorrect] Patients with advanced dementia often have severe problems with activities of daily living and are unable to care for themselves.
C: The patient has pseudodementia. [Incorrect] Pseudodementia is a condition seen in the depressed elderly patients that appear to have dementia. The dementia symptoms resolve in these patients when the dementia is treated.
D: The patient has multi-infarct dementia. [Incorrect] Patients with multi-infarct dementia develop a stepwise decline in cognitive function.
E: The patient's forgetfulness is most likely transient and will resolve over time. [Incorrect] The patient's symptoms are consistent with normal aging and are not likely to resolve over time.

9. C

A: Auditory hallucination [Incorrect] A hallucination is a false sensory perception (for example, hearing voices when alone).
B: Delusion [Incorrect] A delusion is a false belief that is not shared by others (for example, thinking that the FBI is following you).
C: Idea of reference [Correct] The patient demonstrates a false belief that he is being referred to by another person.
D: Illusion [Incorrect] An illusion is a misperception of a real external stimuli (for example, interpreting a pair of shoes sticking out from under the bed as feet).
E: Visual hallucination [Incorrect] A hallucination is a false sensory perception (for example, seeing something that is not really present).

10. D

A: Nightmare disorder. [Incorrect] Patients with nightmare disorder have repetitive frightening nightmares that awaken the patient from sleep. Patients with this disorder are able to remember the nightmares.
B: Nocturnal myoclonus. [Incorrect] Nocturnal myoclonus is characterized by nighttime awakenings and repetitive muscle contractions in the legs. This condition is most common in the elderly.
C: No sleep disorder. [Incorrect] The patient has sleep terror disorder.
D: Sleep terror disorder. [Correct] The vignette describes sleep terror disorder.
E: Temporal lobe epilepsy. [Incorrect] Development of sleep terror disorder during adolescence may be a sign of temporal lobe epilepsy.

11. B

A: Cognitive disturbances [Incorrect] Cognitive disturbances are a negative symptom.

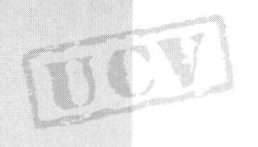

B: Delusions [Correct] Delusions are a positive symptom. Other positive symptoms include hallucinations, strange behavior, talkativeness, and loose associations.
C: Flattened affect [Incorrect] Flattened affect is a negative symptom.
D: Poor grooming [Incorrect] Poor grooming is a negative symptom.
E: Social withdrawal [Incorrect] Social withdrawal is a negative symptom.
F: Thought blocking [Incorrect] Thought blocking is a negative symptom.

12. D

A: Dental caries [Incorrect] Dental caries are common in patients with bulimia nervosa secondary to vomiting.
B: Electrolyte disturbances [Incorrect] Electrolyte disturbances are more common in patients with bulimia nervosa secondary to vomiting.
C: From a low socioeconomic group [Incorrect] Patients with anorexia are most often from a high socioeconomic group.
D: High academic achievement [Correct] Patients with anorexia nervosa are likely to be perfectionist and have high academic achievement. They are often from a high socioeconomic group, exercise excessively, and have abnormal eating habits.
E: Swelling of parotid and salivary glands [Incorrect] Swelling of the parotid and salivary glands are common in patients with bulimia nervosa secondary to vomiting.

13. D

A: Women successfully commit suicide four times more often than men. [Incorrect] Men successfully commit suicide three times more often than women.
B: Approximately 75% of people who attempt suicide once will try again. [Incorrect] About 30% of people who attempt suicide will attempt it again.
C: The suicide rate in the U.S. is about 50 per 100,000. [Incorrect] The U.S. suicide rate is about 12 per 100,000.
D: Suicide is the eighth leading cause of death. [Correct] This statement is true. Suicide follows heart disease, cancer, accidents, stroke, diabetes, pneumonia, and liver cirrhosis.
E: There are about four times more suicide attempts than actual suicides. [Incorrect] There are about nine times more suicide attempts than actual suicides.

14. D

A: Prescribe Haldol. [Incorrect] Haldol is an antipsychotic. It is not indicated in anxiety.

111

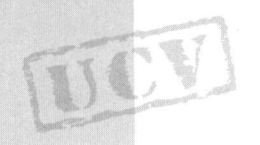

B: Prescribe Wellbutrin. [Incorrect] Wellbutrin is well known to be an effective medication in reliving anxiety, but it does not take effect immediately. Another medication is needed that has an immediate effect.
C: Prescribe Lorazepam initially, then Haldol. [Incorrect] If Haldol is not indicated alone, it would not be indicated in conjunction with another medication.
D: Prescribe Lorazepam initially, then Wellbutrin. [Correct] Both benzodiazepines and Wellbutrin work for anxiety. Lorazepam has an immediate effect, but should only be used for a short time. Wellbutrin takes a few weeks before it is effective and can be used indefinitely. Therefore, they should be used together.
E: Prescribe ECT. [Incorrect] ECT is indicated for severe depression, which the patient does not have.

15. B

A: Major depressive disorder [Incorrect] Patients with major depressive disorder have episodes of depression, but no episodes of mania (elevated mood). This patient clearly exhibits manic episodes.
B: Bipolar I disorder [Correct] Bipolar I disorder is characterized by episodes of mania and depression. This patient clearly exhibits both.
C: Bipolar II disorder [Incorrect] Bipolar II disorder is characterized by hypomanic episodes, in which the elevated mood is not nearly as severe and bipolar I disorder; it is also characterized by depressive episodes as well.
D: Cyclothymic disorder [Incorrect] This disorder is a milder form of bipolar disorder; often times these patients have relatives with a diagnosis of bipolar.
E: Dysthymic disorder [Incorrect] These patients exhibit symptoms of consistent mild depression for at least 2 consecutive years.

16. D

A: 0.81 [Incorrect] Relative risk and attributable risk are used in cohort studies to examine disease risks. Attributable risk (AR) is disease risk in exposed group (E) minus disease risk in unexposed group (U). Relative risk (RR) is disease risk in exposed group/disease risk in unexposed group. In equation form AR=E−U, RR=E/U. We are given that U=0.01. Thus, E=AR+U=0.90+0.01=0.91. RR=0.91/0.01=91. This answer can likely be eliminated even without knowledge of the formulas, because it would mean that exposure to the toxin would make the individuals healthier.
B: 9 [Incorrect] This is a tempting answer, because 0.9/0.01=9. On the real USMLE, they will often play similar formula games, trying to guess what someone would use if they didn't really know.
C: 90 [Incorrect] This is an attempt to make numbers confusing.

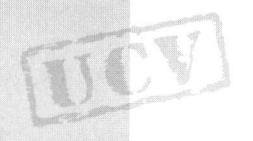

D: 91 [Correct] When there are three that are very similar and another that is similar to one of the three, this can either be a distracter or the right answer. In this case, it is the correct answer.
E: 900 [Incorrect] This is an attempt to make numbers confusing.

17. C

A: Adjustment disorder [Incorrect] There is nothing to indicate that a stressful life event has occurred leading to adjustment disorder.
B: Generalized anxiety disorder [Incorrect] This patient has no indication of anxiety.
C: Obsessive-compulsive disorder [Correct] This patient clearly has recurrent feelings and thoughts, i.e., obsessions regarding cleanliness and germs. This patient also has compulsions including hand washing and cleaning.
D: Panic disorder [Incorrect] Patients with panic disorder have episodic periods of intense anxiety. They are usually sudden in onset, the patient has a feeling of impending doom, and the attacks usually last about 30 minutes.
E: Social phobia [Incorrect] The above patient does not seem to have a fear of social or environmental situations.

18. B

A: Psychotic patients cannot participate in research experiments. [Incorrect] In order to give informed consent, a patient must be aware of the risks, benefits, alternatives, and give consent nor under duress. Psychosis does not prevent giving informed consent unless the psychosis interferes with her ability to understand.
B: Psychotic patients can participate in research experiments. [Correct] The patient seems to have adequate understanding.
C: Being psychotic bears no relation to participation in research protocols. [Incorrect] Being psychotic brings special questions to the question of participating in research protocols.
D: Her family should be consulted for permission. [Incorrect] The patient's family does not have rights to allow her to participate or not participate in research, as she is a competent adult.
E: The patient should be convinced to leave her house for treatment. [Incorrect] This answer does not answer the question.

19. C

A: 4 [Incorrect] Children who are 4 and 5 will say that the amounts of water are different.
B: 5 [Incorrect] Children who are 4 and 5 will say that the amounts of water are different.
C: 6 [Correct] Children who are 6 and 7 know that there is the same amount of water no matter what shape it is in.

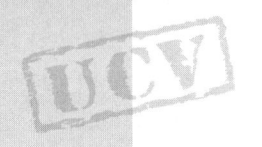

D: 7 [Incorrect] Six is the first age where this behavior is seen.
  E: 8 [Incorrect] By this age, a child should have progressed beyond understanding of mere conservation to understanding of addition and subtraction.

20. D

  A: Doing PSA tests for all men at the VA hospital [Incorrect]. This is secondary care, trying to detect disease at an early stage of that disease.
  B: Doing yearly Pap smears [Incorrect]. This is secondary care, trying to detect disease at an early stage of that disease.
  C: Giving antihypertensive medication to someone with hypertension [Incorrect]. This is tertiary care, designed to reduce disability from a disease.
  D: Giving MMR vaccination to a child [Correct]. Primary care is used to prevent disease occurrence.
  E: Testing a diabetic for peripheral neuropathy [Incorrect]. This is tertiary care, designed to reduce disability from a disease.